MEDICINE

THE ART OF HEALING

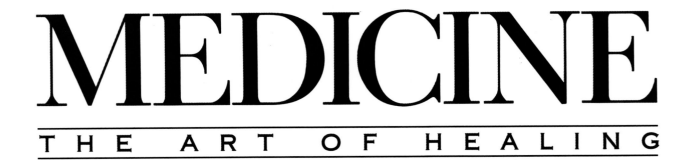

MEDICINE
THE ART OF HEALING

SHERWIN B. NULAND

HUGH LAUTER LEVIN ASSOCIATES, INC.

*Distributed by Macmillan Publishing Company,
New York*

For Molly,
who loves pictures—and loves words even more.

From, Daddy

Copyright © 1992,
Hugh Lauter Levin Associates, Inc.

Design by Kathleen Herlihy-Paoli

Typeset by
U.S. Lithograph, typographers, New York City

Printed in Hong Kong

ISBN 0-88363-292-6

Jacket illustration: Adelbert Seligmann. *Theodor Billroth Operating*. 1890.
Osterreichische Galerie, Vienna.

Frontispiece: Robert C. Hinckley
Detail from *First Operation Under Ether*. 1881–1894.
Boston Medical Library, Francis A. Countway Library of Medicine, Boston

CONTENTS

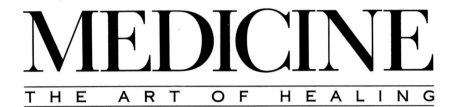

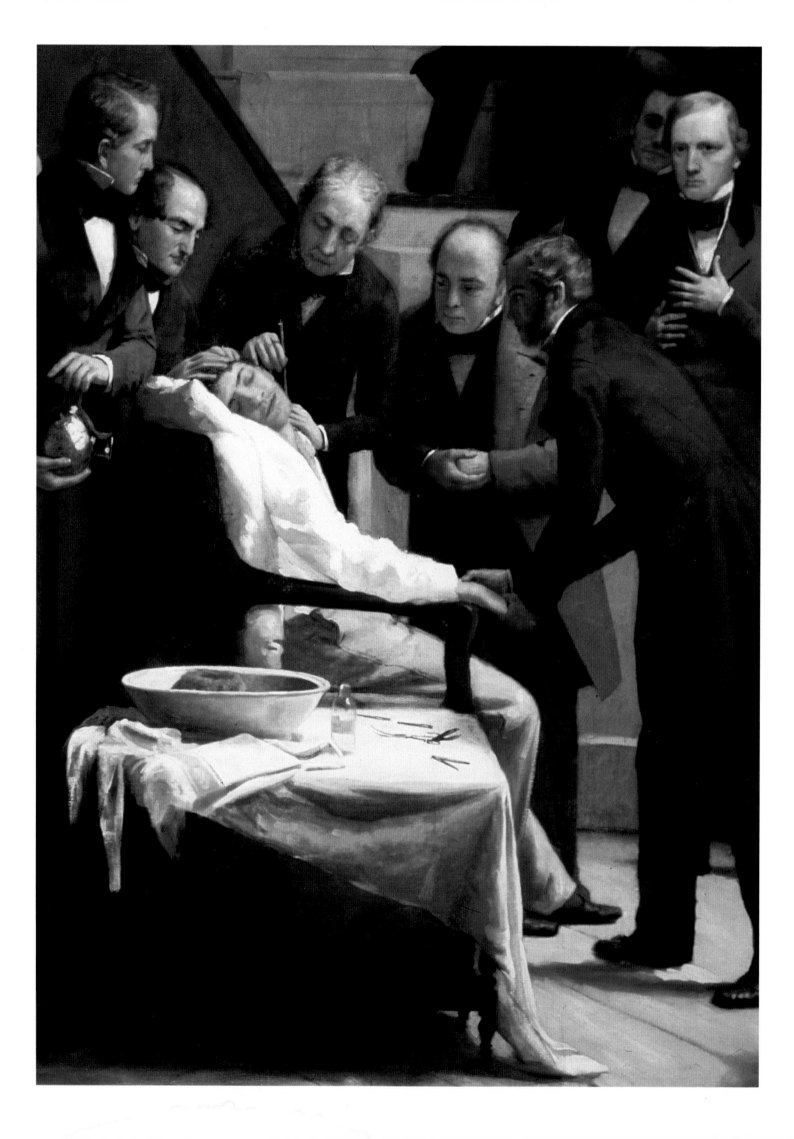

This book is not a history of medicine, and it is not a history of art. While it is more than a picture book of medical progress, it would not be the chosen text of someone seeking a major new contribution to scholarship. There are some new insights, but no radical reinterpretations. Least of all do these pages deliver an encyclopedic reference work for those who would delve into details of the ways in which the visual arts and the healing arts have contributed to each other's development. Everyone who reads this volume will recognize that the fields of human endeavor it embraces are not being explored to the utmost.

In enumerating the various things this book is not, I am making a deliberately transparent attempt to avoid pigeonholing it. None of us —author, editors, consultants, publisher—was quite sure, when we began our exploration, what we would end up with. Having now finished, we are only a little closer to defining our work than we were at first.

But we need not categorize. It should suffice to describe the many facets of this volume, its pictures and texts. Essentially, what we present here is a cavalcade of medical images with great appeal—that is, we have worked in the hope that, for a variety of reasons which the texts make evident, they will appeal to those who enjoy words and pictures just for the pleasures of reading and looking. Were we gastronomically inclined, we would list *Medicine: The Art of Healing* as a smorgasbord—for us, it has been a feast.

Since the very beginnings of the profession of healing, observers of the medical scene, including doctors, have used the powers that are inherent in artistic expression, and they have done so in many different ways. Art, as didactic illustration, is a vehicle for the transmission of knowledge: there is a type of art that serves as social commentary; there is art as historic documentation; art as an expression of value; art as a statement of religious faith; art as portraiture; art as a jeremiad; art as encomium; art as metaphor; art as depiction of universal experience; art to disperse the demons of fear.

Art is as timeless as it is wordless. In this it differs from medical science, which is ever a creature uniquely of and for its time and has always required a literal articulation to be fully understood. Perhaps these very differences explain why two such seemingly disparate manifestations of culture should so naturally complement each other. Art and medicine belong together, and we who have enjoyed demonstrating their affinity hope that this book, if it does nothing else, will serve to convey the immense pleasure that comes from contemplating the results of that melding.

Except for our determination to provide a panorama of history, there have been only two criteria used in the process of selecting the works of art for this volume. The first was singular for the picture itself: sometimes a picture was chosen to illustrate a particular genre of art, sometimes a particular genre of science. Some of the pictures have been chosen for their beauty alone, and some for their content alone. A few of the pictures are famous, and a few are so obscure that the average reader would have difficulty tracking them down. The same may be said about the artists, several of whom are in fact unknown.

The second criterion was singular for the author, actually so singular that it might be termed idiosyncratic: each of the pictures that appears in this book has been chosen because it is one of those that *I* think is important, that *I* enjoy looking at, and that *I* have studied with profit. If these prove to be sentiments shared by many readers, *I*, among those associated with *Medicine: The Art of Healing*, will be the most gratified.

The selection begins with images that evoke the origins of Western concepts of healing. Hippocrates lived during the golden period of Greek civilization, the age of Pericles. Socrates, Plato, Aristotle, Aeschylus, Sophocles, and Herodotus were alive during some or all of Hippocrates' almost one hundred years. (He died about a decade before Alexander the Great was born.) To Hippocrates and his followers we owe the foundations of the clinical principles and the ethics that grew, albeit through long periods of stagnation and irregular progression, into modern medical science. The famous Oath of Hippocrates is still recited during medical school graduations at many Western universities. No matter that historical research has established that the writings attributed to him are really the work of many authors over a period of several hundred pre-Christian years, Hippocrates remains enshrined as the Father of Medicine.

Galen, the Greek healer and researcher who was the foremost physician of the Roman Empire, justifiably considered himself Hippocrates' rightful heir. He expanded and codified the Hippocratic doctrines and introduced experimentation into the study of healing, but so authoritarian and imperious was he that his dogmatic opinions were not seriously challenged for some fourteen hundred years. When the Moslems founded their nation and became the dominant force in medicine, they took Galen unto themselves; they were as devoted in their belief in him as they were to the new religion they rapidly spread through the Arabian Peninsula, North Africa, and Europe. With medical theory becoming fixed on the model of Galenism, the art of healing became enmired in the Greek system in which most disease was thought to be caused by imbalances of bodily fluids—blood, phlegm, yellow bile, and black bile—called humors.

Nevertheless, a modicum of progress was made during the almost fourteen hundred post-Galenic years in the more practical hands-on technical aspects of surgery. Several important texts appeared in which were to be found graphic descriptions, appropriately illustrated, of wound treatment, hernia surgery, bladder-stone removal, and rectal operations. Of the master *chirurgeons*, or surgeons, of the Middle Ages, we show here two examples of the most renowned, Henri de Mondeville and John of Arderne. This is art as didactic illustration, meant for the transmission of knowledge.

Even for the rough-and-ready chirurgical artisans of the time (perhaps *especially* for them), instruction on ethical behavior was mandatory, and respected authorities like Henri and John did not hesitate to teach their readers the behavior expected of those who would call themselves surgeons. Their writings provide interesting and even amusing insights for today's readers, and several of Henri's injunctions have been included in our book.

Medicine awoke from its long torpor during the Renaissance, as did so many other areas of European culture. Though not a physician, the great Leonardo da Vinci led the way with his dissections and drawings of every aspect of human anatomy. His more than seven hundred fifty anatomic sketches were lost and in fact forgotten within a generation of his death, but in his day they seem to have exerted a substantial influence on artists and anatomists. Not until the sketches were rediscovered in 1898 was the magnitude of Leonardo's understanding of the human body fully appreciated. Done in red chalk, they represent the first accurate images in existence of actual dissections.

The great artists of the Renaissance—Michelangelo, Raphael, Titian, Dürer, and others—were not slow to follow. Their magnificent paintings and sculptures demonstrate the assiduous attention they paid to their personal experience of dissection. The result was a rebirth of interest in the details of the human body's structure. No longer would the old Galenic anatomy be acceptable, based as it was on the study of dogs and monkeys. *Of the Structure of the Human Body (De humani corporis fabrica)* is, in fact, the title of the book that heralded acceptance of the change. It was written by Andreas Vesalius, a Belgian anatomist who, at twenty-eight, was already a professor at the University of Padua.

The dissections of Vesalius, as drawn by Titian's pupil Stephen van Calcar, quickly became the standard for accurate observation and for the objective analysis of the evidences of a medical researcher's five senses. Medicine began to throw off the Galenic yoke, at least in the approach to theory: belief in the four humors would continue to influence therapy for three more centuries.

Another influence was the power of religious faith. The early Christian church appropriated many of the principles of Greek medicine into its healing mission and added to them the belief in divine intervention. Jesus thus replaced Aesculapius, the god of healing, and even overshadowed Hippocrates. Though the latter was the most well-known leader of a school that abjured belief in the supernatural, in both the cause and the treatment of sickness, his teachings are manifest, ironically, in medieval Christian images of healing. This book contains the reproduction of a twelfth-century manuscript in which the Oath of Hippocrates is written in the shape of a cross.

Raffaello Sanzio, or Raphael, in his depiction of the transfiguration of Jesus, has shown the divine healing of an epileptic child in the presence of the apostles Peter, James, and John, high on a mountain that might have been Mount Tabor. During the Renaissance, many immortal images were created in the name of art as a statement of religious faith, but in relation to healing there is not one whose magnificence equals Raphael's masterpiece. Even William Hogarth was inspired by the healing miracles of Jesus, leaving aside his usual documentary satirical style to create *The Pool of Bethesda*.

Among the miracles attributed to the saints were prodigious feats of healing, but none has more greatly captured the imaginations of modern surgeons, particularly transplant surgeons, than the transplanting of a leg by the brothers Cosmas and Damian. The scene has appeared in the works of a number of artists, and one fine representation of it has been chosen for this book.

During the late Middle Ages and the Renaissance, even in the midst of an all-encompassing belief in God's power to afflict and to heal, events of medical and cultural enormity were overtaking Europe in the forms of epidemics and wars. The terrors of pestilence—plague, cholera, and syphilis—enveloped the populace of every Western country. Physicians were impotent in the face of such overwhelming diseases. Painters documented the devastation, sometimes objectively and sometimes with the theme of punishment and penitence—art as historic documentation, art as jeremiad, art as metaphor.

Every natural disaster finally comes to an end, and so it was with the great epidemics. Yet the diseases remained quietly endemic until the twentieth century, ready to flare up anywhere and at any time. Medical progress continued, not in any steady upward course, but rather in fits and starts, not always recognized, appreciated, or utilized.

The seventeenth century saw the introduction of inductive reasoning and therefore of true experimental science as we know it today. The earliest benefit to medicine of the methods of scientific research was the discovery of the circulation of the blood by William Harvey in 1628. Artists began to see medical researchers in a new light: they were men who were uncovering the secrets of nature, with the aim of healing their fellows. In Robert Hannah's *William Harvey Presenting a Deer Heart to His King*, in Rembrandt's portrayal of Dr. Tulp, in Sir Joshua Reynolds's portrait of a contemplative John Hunter, we see art not only as portraiture, but as encomium. Even

in caricature, doctors were often lauded. When *Vanity Fair*'s "Spy" drew his cartoon of Rudolf Virchow, he meant it as a statement of the German scientist's preeminence over the medical thinking of the late nineteenth century.

It was not invariably so. While the most revered of the physicians were being depicted as intellectual icons, the general run of medical men were often lampooned as venal, mendacious charlatans, more interested in purse than in patient. There seems to have been good reason for this. Although there were a few professional societies and some laws that regulated the behavior of physicians, it was not difficult in the seventeenth, eighteenth, and even the nineteenth century, to call oneself a doctor of one variety or another and go out to fleece the unwary. The toothpullers and uroscopists are but two of the varieties of quackery and showmanship that bedevilled unsuspecting patients in those days. Even the real doctors, poorly trained as most of them were, were all too often unable to offer their patients anything but the diarrhea of calomel, the blistering of plasters, and the exhaustion of bloodletting.

No wonder, then, that the medical profession became an appropriate target for caricaturists such as Thomas Rowlandson and James Gillray in England and, later, Honoré Daumier in France, who found plenty of "warts" to poke fun at. Sometimes the doctors must have felt as though the tables had been turned and that the bloodletting lancets were being used on them. Here we have art as social commentary.

Diseases, too, were caricatured, as though ridiculing their ravages would somehow demystify them and take away their power to frighten. This is art to disperse the demons of fear. Cholera, headache, melancholia, gout, and other ailments were cartooned in some of the most popular satirical images of the day. Gillray's *Gout* has endured precisely because of its savage accuracy. Send-ups of gout were welcomed by a wide audience, other than the victims themselves, because the malady was perceived as a curse visited on the moneyed classes in retribution for their self-indulgent lives. Interestingly, there are no caricatures of cancer.

Even while there was plenty of reason to ridicule physicians, the various branches of the profession continued their often uneven advances in regulating themselves, trying to provide better methods and facilities for healing. Hans Holbein's depiction of Henry VIII approving the union between barbers and surgeons is an illustration of a quiet yet important step forward in the professionalization of at least one medical specialty. This is art as historic documentation, in which time is stopped in its tracks to record an important scene for posterity. The painting of St. John's Hospital at Bruges, Belgium, is another such example, as is Robert Hinckley's almost photographic representation of the morning of October 16, 1846, when ether was first demonstrated as a surgical anesthetic. The same might be said of the deathbed scene of George Washington. Such art easily slips into portraiture, especially when the subject is a renowned figure of his time, such as Guillaume Dupuytren, John Hunter, or Samuel Gross. The paintings of the latter two are not only portraits; each picture appears also to be an encomium created by an admiring artist. Sir Joshua Reynolds, who did the Hunter painting, was actually his subject's neighbor. Andrew Wyeth, who painted a salutation to his son's pediatrician, Margaret Handy, was also that doctor's close friend.

The word *doctor* derives from the Latin *docere*, which means teacher. The Hippocratic Oath enjoins the newly sworn physician to take on as disciples those "who have signed the covenant and have taken an oath according to the law of medicine," and "to teach them this Art." Medicine thus combines two of the highest callings, to heal and to teach. Not surprisingly, teaching is a common theme in depictions of medical life. Fully a quarter of the illustrations in this volume came from textbooks and manuscripts written for the purpose of instruction. Another eight are in one form or another portraits of great medical teachers. John Singer Sargent's *The Four Doctors* is a formal sitting of a quartet of the greatest medical pedagogues our country has ever produced. Two of our illustrations, done half a millennium apart, are scenes that contrast classroom methods whereby students familiarize themselves with the human body.

A brief introduction such as this cannot describe all the illustrations chosen for the following pages, and it only touches upon the various ways in which artists have used medical themes. The texts and pictures will remedy these limitations, however, and probably bring other possibilities to mind. Not to go unmentioned is a point of similarity between the method of the artist and the method of the healer. Each is, after all, first an observer, then an interpreter, and then a synthesizer. When the artist has synthesized his observations, impressions, experience, and particular world view, he knows how to create his picture or statue. When a physician has synthesized his observations, impressions, experience, and particular world view, he arrives at a diagnosis and knows how to create his therapy. Perhaps this is one of the reasons that medicine will always be an Art.

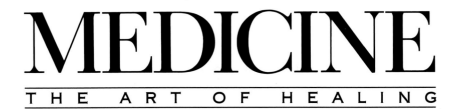

MEDICINE

THE ART OF HEALING

Twelfth century

During the decline of the Roman Empire, the center of European culture was transferred to the East. As the heritage of Greek and Roman civilization fell under the authority of Byzantine Christianity, patterns of medical thought were profoundly affected. Most obvious was a change in direction from an objective gathering of observations and conclusions toward a system based on religious faith.

Henceforth, the sick and those who would care for them were to be dependent on divine benevolence. The care of the sick became a Christian duty, not only for individuals, but also for the community as a whole. Perhaps the most direct statement of this philosophy is to be found in the fifth chapter of the epistle of St. James: "Is any sick among you? Let him call for the elders of the church; and let them pray over him, anointing him with oil in the name of the Lord."

Hospitals and hospices flourished, the art of nursing built its foundations, and the great tradition of Christian charity to the disabled spread over every area controlled by the ecclesiastics. For the faithful, the power of religious medicine was strengthened by prayer, the laying-on of hands, unction, miracles, and the lives of saints, a number of whom were invoked as protection against certain diseases or because of a specific miraculous cure. Some of the most renowned Christian physicians of the Byzantine period were priests and bishops who preached the charity of Christ as the ultimate force in healing.

In spite of its many beneficial effects, a medicine founded on faith and on church dogma is unlikely to make major contributions to understanding the biological processes of disease. The entire Byzantine period was, in fact, a stagnant era for medical progress. Not until the Renaissance would medicine free itself from the constrictions imposed on it by ecclesiastical authority. Ironically, when progress began again it would be that same ecclesiastical authority that would recognize the need to seek once more for scientific truths. It was with the sanction of Renaissance popes, bishops, and priests that the reawakening of medicine began after a thousand post-Roman years.

The dominance of religion over medical thought resulted in some peculiar manifestations, as the worship of Aesculapius, the Greek god of healing, gave way to a worship of Christ. One example of this is the way in which some of the early images of Christ were modeled upon the traditional face of Aesculapius. Statues of Aesculapius were venerated in some of the early churches as though they were really statues of Jesus. In that era of reliance on dictates from high places, the influence of Hippocrates and Galen became strengthened, as though the two Greek physicians had been adopted by the Church and made canonical authorities. No wonder, then, that there is to be found in the Vatican Library a twelfth-century manuscript in which the Oath of Hippocrates is written in the form of a cross. Even the Father of Medicine, among whose legacies was the separation of healing from divine or supernatural intervention, had been converted posthumously into a Christian.

Colorplate 1. Byzantine manuscript. Vatican Biblioteca Apostolica, Rome.

λόγου· ἀπὸ τῶν προειρημένων. ὅτι μὲν ἡμῖν ἀρημόμεθα· ὑπὲρ ταῦτα καταπαύσω· τῷ δὲ
δὲ προτέρους ἡμετέρους καὶ τοῖς ἡμιν ολοιπεῖς ιδιομενος εῖναι. καὶ θεῶν
καὶ πρὸς τῶν ερεκα· καὶ χαρίτων· ἀ ἀπ᾿ ἀνθρώποις παρ ανθρωπων γίνονται· ἄρα
με τ εχριν τα αλλα θρημαο· εἰς δὲ φιλανθρωπα τρεπεσθαι· εἰ γαρ μεν τι
ἡμετέρα πολει τουτο αρχωτα ζομεθα· οὐ καὶ ὁ δ᾿ πονειδοντες· ὡριμ
εομεθ ακυρησομεν :·

─────────────

Ἐκ τοῦ κατὰ τὸν Ἱπποκράτην ὅρκου
καθ᾿ ὅσον οἷόν τε Χριστιανῶν ὄντα·
Εὐλογητὸς ὁ Θεὸς καὶ πατὴρ τοῦ κυρίου ἡμῶν
Ἰησοῦ Χριστοῦ, ὁ ὢν εὐλογητὸς εἰς τοὺς αἰ-
ῶνας· οὐ καταψεύσομαι· ὁμολο-
γῶ τὴν τῆς ἰατρικῆς τέχνην ἀσκεῖν
βιοτήν· οὐ δὲ δώσω οὐδενὶ αἰτη-
θεὶς φάρμακον θανάσιμον· οὐδὲ
ὑφηγήσομαι ξυμβουλίην τοιήνδε·
ὁμοίως δὲ οὐδὲ γυναικὶ ξύσσον

φθόριον· ἁγνῶς δὲ καὶ ὁσίως διατηρήσω βίον τε τὸν ἐμὸν καὶ τέχνην τὴν ἐμὴν· οὐ
τεμέω δὲ οὐδὲ μὴν λιθιῶντας· ἀλλὰ παραχωρήσω ἐργάτησιν ἀνδράσι πρήξιος τῆσδε. ἐς
οἰκίας δὲ ὁκόσας ἂν ἐσίω, ἐσελεύσομαι ἐπ᾿ ὠφελείῃ καμνόντων· ἐκτὸς ἐὼν πάσης ἀδικίης
ἑκουσίης τε καὶ φθορίης τῆς τε ἄλλης καὶ ἀφρο-
δισίων ἔργων ἐπί τε γυναικείων σωμάτων καὶ ἀν-
δρείων, ἐλευθέρων τε καὶ δούλων· ἃ δ᾿ ἂν ἐν θερα-
πείῃ ἢ ἴδω ἢ ἀκούσω ἢ ἄνευ θεραπείης οὐ
κατὰ τὸν βίον ἀνθρώπων ἃ μὴ χρή ποτε
ἐκλαλεῖσθαι ἔξω σιγήσομαι, ἄρρητα
ἡγεύμενος εἶναι τὰ τοιαῦτα· ὅρκον μὲν
οὖν μοι τόνδε ἐπιτελέα ποιοῦν-
τι καὶ μὴ ξυγχέοντι εἴη ἐπαύρασθαι
καὶ βίου καὶ τέχνης δοξαζο-
μένῳ παρὰ πᾶσιν ἀνθρώποις
εἰς τὸν ἅπαντα χρόνον· εἰ δ᾿ ὁρκοῦντι
μοι ναί· εἴη δέ μοι ·

τέλος

1314

Henri de Mondeville

In a time when wounds were believed to require the presence of pus in order to heal, Henri de Mondeville knew better; in a time when almost all surgeons were poorly trained artisans without formal education, Henri de Mondeville was one of the *medicins-chirurgiens*, who had graduated from a medical school with the degree of Master, a title held in the same esteem as a physician's doctorate; in a time when a knowledge of the body's structure was considered to be of little use in the practical treatment of disease, Henri de Mondeville lectured in anatomy at the medical school of the University of Montpellier.

Henri began his great surgical treatise *Chirurgie* in 1306 and continued to work on it for ten years, even after it had been translated from its original Latin into French in 1314, in order to make it widely comprehensible to surgeons. The first of its five treatises, dealing with anatomy, has thirteen illustrations in color, including drawings of original dissections. The frontispiece of the 1314 manuscript is reproduced here, showing de Mondeville lecturing from a Latin text and wearing a gown tailored in an ecclesiastical manner.

The second and third treatises in *Chirurgie* deal with wounds and surgical problems. Henri rejected the contemporary practice of probing wounds and applying ointments and poultices—treatments that encouraged inflammation and infection. In his words: "Many more surgeons know how to produce pus than to heal a wound." He was almost modern in his insistence on cleanliness and the removal of injured tissue, lest it add to the infection. After washing the wound clean, he stitched it as soon as possible and did not use the common potions of the day, which were meant to promote healing by scar formation: "We call [healing] 'first intention' because nature will always do better if it is left unhindered, and the surgeon, who is nature's imitator, should try to heal all wounds in all parts of the body in the same way."

Henri believed that surgeons should be trained as physicians, a wishful thought that would not become a reality until more than five hundred years after his death. His writings abound in advice on the proper behavior of a surgeon toward both patients and colleagues. Sometimes he recommended that the healer wage psychological warfare against disease: "Keep up your patient's spirits by music of viols and ten-stringed psaltery, or by forged letters describing the death of his enemies, or by telling him that he has been elected to a bishopric, if a churchman."

Henri de Mondeville had no qualms about discussing fees, and his wryly pragmatic advice has been a source of admiration and amusement alike: "The surgeon should give the poor gratuitous care; if possible the rich should pay well." And, in another place: "Never dine with a patient who is in your debt, but get your dinner at an inn, otherwise he will deduct his hospitality from your fee."

Colorplate 2. Illuminated manuscript. Bibliotheque Nationale, Paris.

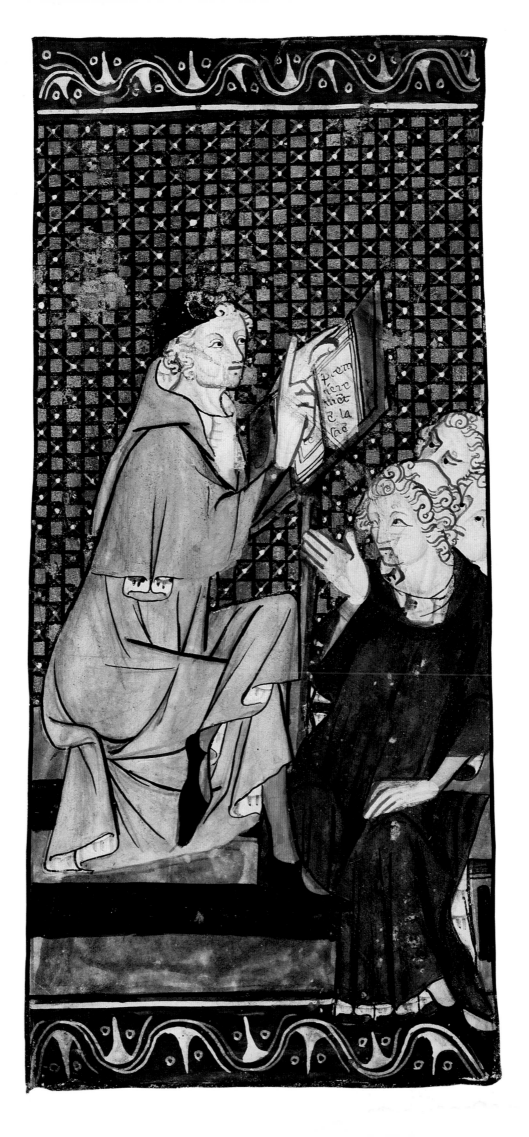

ca. 1390

The tradition of that type of medical text called the herbal is rooted, as it were, in classical practices not only of the West but also of Chinese and Indian cultures. In its simplest form, an herbal is a compilation of information about those plants that have medical uses. Certainly the best known among the earliest of the Western herbals is *De materia medica*, written by Dioscorides, a Greek surgeon in the army of the Roman emperor Nero. This work served as a foundation for the pharmacopeia for at least a millennium and a half from the time it was written in the first century A.D. The work illustrated here is from *Tacuinum sanitatis in medicina*, one of the great medieval herbals that included dramatic depictions of certain characteristics of the botanicals that the text described. Written in northern Italy around 1390, this illuminated codex provides some interesting examples of the magical qualities that many people in the Middle Ages associated with pharmacologically active plants.

Because the mandrake (*Mandragora officinarum*) has a forked root, it requires only a bit of imagination to see it as the lower half of a human body. For this reason, it was used as a love potion and is, in fact, still valued in certain parts of the world for its supposed ability to aid in conception.

In a similar sort of folk tradition, another characteristic was attributed to the humanoid plant: it was believed capable of emitting a shriek of such terrifying quality that it might kill anyone who attempted to pull it out of the ground. What we see in the illustration from the *Tacuinum* is a root-cutter using a technique intended to circumvent the death-dealing power. He has tied a rope around the neck of a dog that is to be sacrificed to protect his life. The other end of the rope is attached to the mandrake, so that it will be pulled up when the animal rushes to a bowl of water placed at a sufficient distance. The mandrake is thus harvested, the dog dies, and the root-cutter triumphs.

The mandrake did, in fact, have an important role to play in medicine: the juice obtained from its root and its fruit contains a belladonna-like substance called an alkaloid, which has a narcotic effect similar to that of opium. In *De materia medica*, Dioscorides recommended that it be used by physicians "for such as cannot sleep or are grievously pained, and upon being cut or cauterized, the wish to make a not-feeling pain.... For they do not apprehend the pain, because they are overborne with dead sleep."

Alkaloids derived from the mandrake, from poppies, and from henbane were the commonly used narcotic agents for the agonies of surgery and trauma all through the Greco-Roman, medieval, and Renaissance periods. Even later, up until the invention of anesthesia and new narcotics in the nineteenth century, they continued in use, along with alcohol, as mainstays in the relief of pain.

Colorplate 3. Veronese or Lombard manuscript illustration. 16⅝ × 9⅛″ (33.3 × 23.2 cm). Österreichische Nationalbibliothek, Vienna.

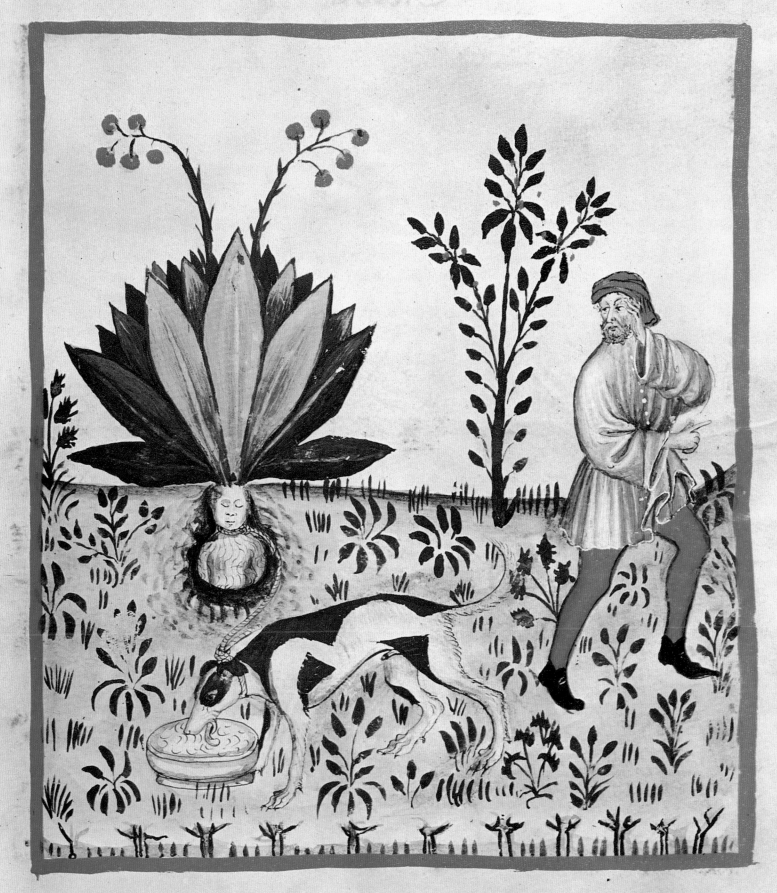

fructus mandragore. opto. fri. in; sic i 2. Electo magni odonfert. muani. odonatio itia sedi.
calam. 7 ugilias. emplando elefintie 7 isectioib; nigris cutis. nocuini. ebetat sensus. Re
nocti. cu fructu edere. Quid gnat no e comestibile; uenit. ca. iuueib; estate 7 mediams.

After 1412

John of Arderne

Unlike most surgeons of his time, John of Arderne was a well-educated man, although he never attended a university. He wrote in Latin, which meant that his surgical colleagues usually required a translation into the vernacular before they could make use of his text. Even without translation, however, the graphic and detailed quality of some of his illustrations enabled his techniques to be understood even by illiterate barbers. His works were widely used for almost two hundred years after he wrote them in the latter part of the fourteenth century.

John acquired much of his training and experience during the course of military campaigns. He served from the mid-1330s to the mid-1340s in the Hundred Years' War and then returned to settle in the city of Newark, in Nottinghamshire. Around 1370, when he was in his early sixties and the proprietor of a large practice, he moved to London and joined the Guild of Military Surgeons. It was here that he began to write of the experiences of his long career.

John was highly regarded by his physician contemporaries, which in itself distinguished him from the surgeons of his time, many of whom were ill-trained barbers who did simple surgical procedures. He proudly referred to himself as *chirurgus inter medicos*, a surgeon among physicians. Nevertheless, neither his surgical skills nor his wide education sufficed to immunize him against the temptation of using superstition as an adjunct to his more direct methods of healing. One of his biographers, Sir D'Arcy Power, has said: "Nothing pleased him more than a charm."

The accompanying plate is part of a large vellum scroll that is a fifteenth-century edition of John's *De arte phisicali et de chirurgia*, now housed at the Royal Library in Stockholm. A crude, almost childlike representation of a cadaver split up the middle and laid open, the picture reflects the general ignorance of anatomy that then existed; this, in turn, reflects the heritage of a millennium of Galenic error.

In the upper portion of the scroll, a surgeon's hand is seen holding the end of a long string. Such strings were used by John in his operation for rectal fistula, a difficult chronic disease in which he successfully specialized at a time when its cure defied most methods of treatment. A fistula is a tunnel-like tract that runs from an opening on the surface of the skin inward to an internal organ, often the rectum; its cause is infection or injury. John's operation consisted of threading a string onto a probe and then passing it from the skin opening into the tract and then through to the rectum. By cutting down onto the string or a shield placed alongside it, he laid open the entire tract, which would then gradually heal from its depth outward. These are the basic principles of the method used to treat this very common disease today.

Colorplate 4. Vellum scroll. 213⅝ × 14³/₁₆" (542.6 × 36 cm). The Royal Library, Stockholm.

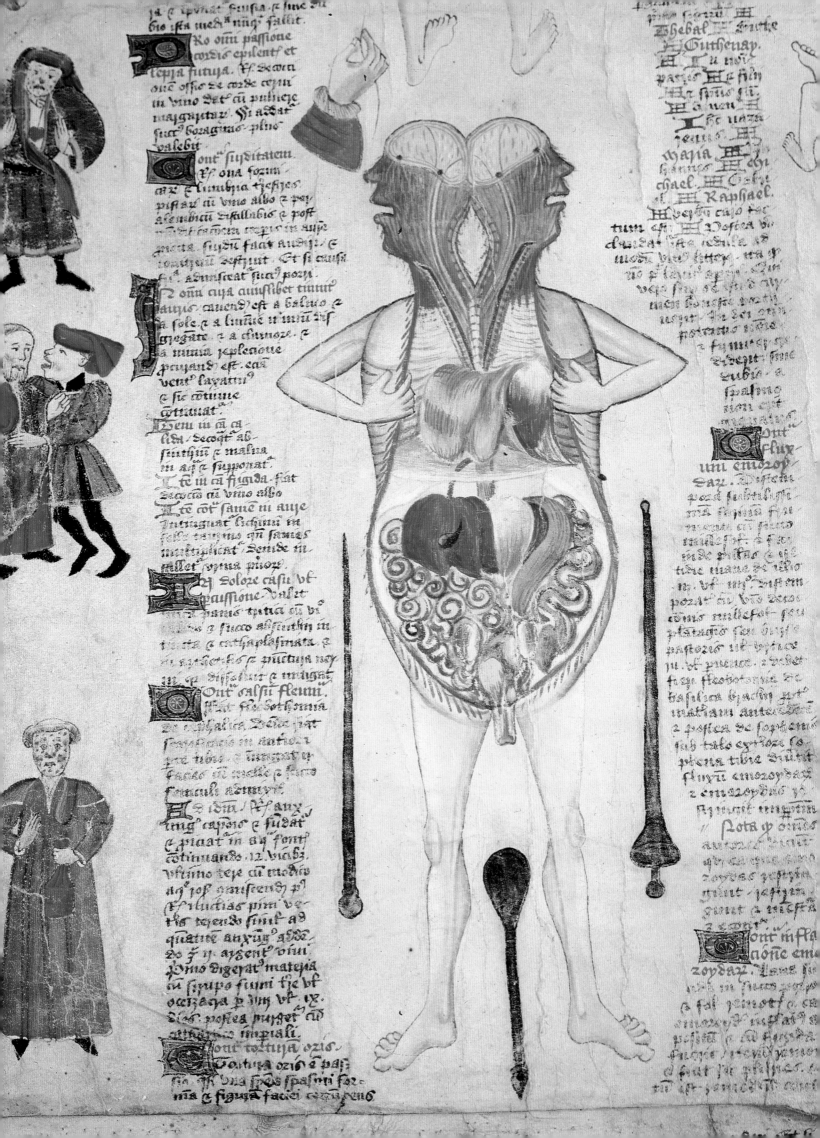

ca. 1440

Avicenna

Avicenna (980–1037), the Persian-born physician and philosopher, was a child prodigy. By the age of ten he had memorized the Koran and a great deal of other Arabic literature as well. While still a teenager he decided to become a physician. To achieve his goal he worked day and night in the indefatigable manner that was to characterize his endeavors for the rest of his life. His mastery of medicine by the age of eighteen becomes all the more remarkable when it is pointed out that he was teaching himself logic, mathematics, and philosophy at the same time.

Although Avicenna wrote many works in the various intellectual fields in which he excelled, his magnum opus was the *Canon of Medicine*, a compendium of all the known teachings of the classical Greek physicians and the Arab writers who followed the Galenic heritage. Although there were many Arab and Jewish medical authors in the Moslem empire—Rhazes, Haly Abbas, Albucasis, Isaac Judaeus, and Maimonides, to mention some of the greatest—the most influential was Avicenna. His *Canon* was the supreme authority in medicine for six centuries, in the Middle East, North Africa, and Europe. As late as 1650, it was still being relied upon as the major text in several European schools, including those of Louvain and Montpellier.

How did it come about that Avicenna replaced Galen, who had dominated medical thought since the third century? When the Moslem Empire burst forth from its Middle Eastern confines in the eighth century, it became ever-expanding in its cultural and scientific energy. The writings of Galen, Oribasius, Alexander of Tralles, and Paul of Agina were translated into Arabic, studied, edited, annotated, and written anew by Moslem and Jewish physicians until these newer works became the commanding body of medical thought of the time. When a Christian doctor of the twelfth or thirteenth century studied medicine, he was usually studying Avicenna translated into Latin. Since the *Canon* was really an edited, interpreted, and expanded version of Galen and Hippocrates, with some Aristotle thrown in (their works were by then lost to the Christian world), Europeans were learning Greek medicine transmitted through a series of translators and redactors. No wonder that many of the original Greek ideas were distorted beyond recognition. It was not until after the Turkish conquest of Constantinople in 1453 that the actual Greek manuscripts of Byzantium found their way back to Europe so that they could be converted directly into Latin. This process resulted in a reawakening of classical learning in Western Europe and a renaissance in medicine led by such as Andreas Vesalius, in the sixteenth century, and William Harvey, in the seventeenth.

The illuminated manuscript shown here is from a fifteenth-century Hebrew edition of Avicenna's *Canon*. Because so many of the leading physicians of the time were Jews whose origins were in the Moslem lands, the works of the authors of all three religions were often translated into Hebrew. The great theologian-physician Rabbi Moses Maimonides, for example, wrote all his medical works in Arabic, and they therefore required later editions in Hebrew.

The central scene is of an open-air pharmacy, and the various panels illustrate several of the routine methods of care, such as bleeding, plasters, and specialized baths.

Colorplate 5. Illuminated manuscript. Biblioteca Universitaria, Bologna.

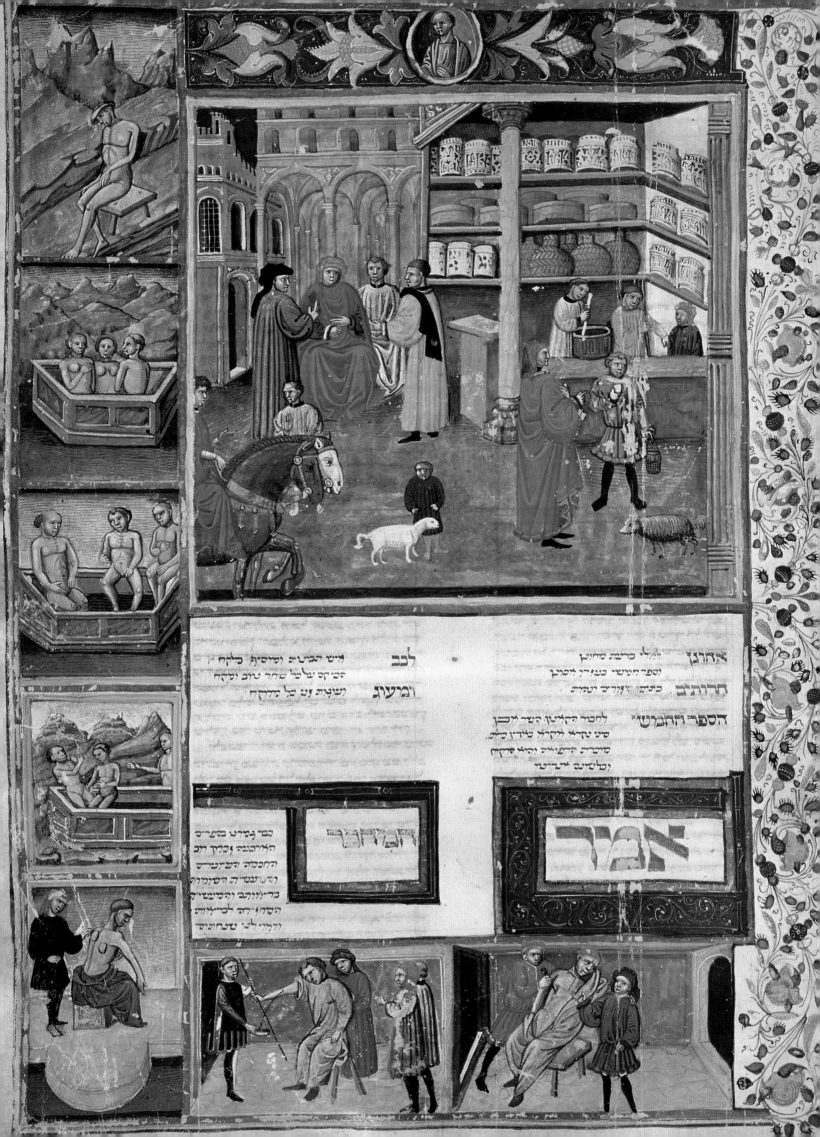

ca. 1472

The self-proclaimed heir of Hippocrates, Galen was the most influential physician of all time. A Greek born in Asia Minor in A.D. 130, he began his medical training in his home city of Pergamon. Later he spent five years studying in the great metropolis of Alexandria. Arriving in Rome at the age of thirty-two, he rapidly established his reputaton as an unusually effective healer and a skilled investigator into the functions of various organs of the body. This he did in a series of ingenious experiments on dogs and monkeys. In the process of his research, he elucidated certain basic principles of physiology that had been poorly understood previously.

By a combination of extraordinary ability and a knack for publicizing himself, Galen established his reputation as a respected authority throughout the Roman Empire, eventually attaining the rank of physician to the emperor Marcus Aurelius. A prolific writer, his works were infused with an air of authority that made him a dominant figure in public life. After his death in A.D. 201, his teachings became the inspiration for all Arabic medical writings and the foundation of European medicine for fifteen hundred years.

The primary theory on which Greek medicine was based was that of the four humors. It was thought that an individual remains healthy so long as four fluids—blood, phlegm, yellow bile, and black bile—remain in a state of equilibrium within the body. Sickness occurs when, for any of a variety of reasons, one of the humors becomes excessive. Although this concept predated Hippocrates, it became refined and codified in the Greek writings, taking on the stature of canonic law in the works of Galen.

Galen believed that not only the state of health but also the basic temperament of any individual is determined by the degree to which one or another of the humors predominates. By this formulation, there are four personality types, as illustrated by this fifteenth-century manuscript. On the upper left, we see a man whose predominant humor is blood; he is therefore sanguine, which in Galenic physiology meant that he had a warm, passionate character. He is appropriately shown serenading a lady, no doubt with more direct manifestations of his passion in mind. The man in the panel to the right is phlegmatic, sluggish, dull; his face is expressionless, and it is with good reason that the lady resists his uninspired overtures. In the bottom left panel, the yellow bile of the choleric man makes him quick to anger, subject to fits of rage. On the other hand, the black bile (Gr. *melas*, 'black'; *chole*, 'bile') of the melancholic man accounts for a depression so deep that he cannot force himself to get out of bed.

Colorplate 6. Illuminated manuscript. 11⅝ × 7⅝" (29.5 × 19.4 cm). Zentralbibliothek, Zurich.

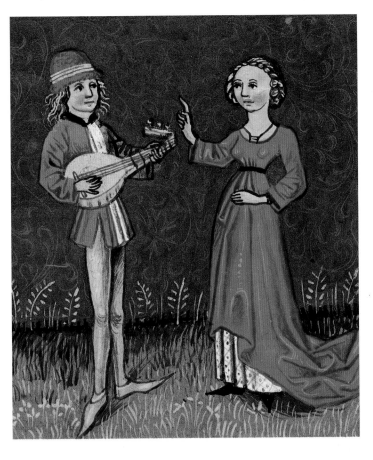

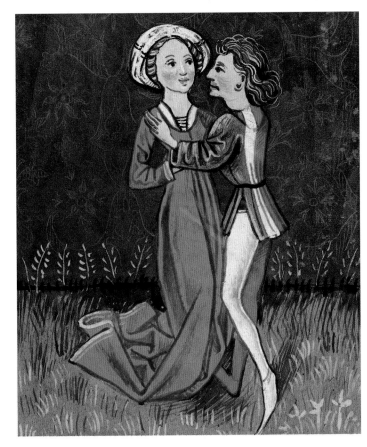

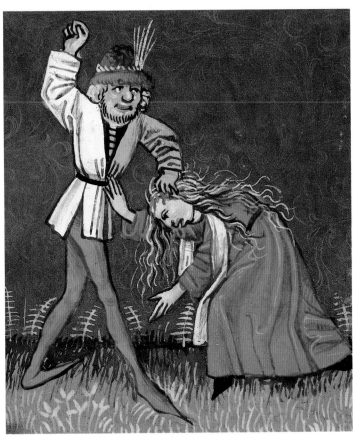

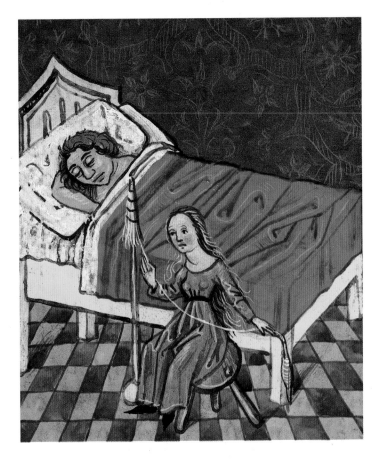

DISSECTION SCENE,
FROM *FASCICULO DI MEDICINA*

1493

Johannes de Ketham

The most conspicuous and certainly the most productive of the collaborations between art and medicine occurred in the late fifteenth and early sixteenth centuries, when the humanism so characteristic of the Renaissance was expressed through a surge of interest in study of the human body. The result would transform both medicine and art; it is not surprising that the names of the famous painters and sculptors of the time are intertwined with the medical history of that era.

Nowhere in Europe was this movement more manifest than in the flourishing cities of northern Italy, particularly in their universities. In 1482, Pope Sixtus IV, who had been a university student in Bologna and Padua, issued a bull that allowed local clergy to permit human dissection. The Prior of the Church of San Spirito in Florence, for example, found it appropriate to grant dissecting privileges to a promising young man named Michelangelo Buonarroti. Such decisions, although beneficial to doctors, were often made for reasons that were hardly disinterested. Churches were beautified, and religious leaders were painted, sculpted, and in other ways honored, by the talents and discoveries of the new breed of dissectors.

A great deal of progress was made in anatomy during this period, as doctors relied increasingly on their own observations and less on the received wisdom, handed down through the centuries, that repeated the errors of Galen. The process culminated in the great contribution of Andreas Vesalius. In 1543, the dissections of Vesalius and the drawings of one of Titian's pupils established the principle that the future of medical progress lay in the accumulation and study of objective, verifiable experiences and in the discarding of principles based only upon the unthinking acceptance of the authority of long-dead sages.

This illustration has long been used by medical historians to describe the pre-Vesalian method of teaching anatomy by rote acceptance of the old treatises. The picture originally appeared in *Fasciculo di medicina*, by Johannes de Ketham, in 1493. The edition included the *Anatomy* of Mondino, an Italian physician who had completed his text in 1316 but had never fully published it. Seated high on his chair (herein lies the origin of *chairman*, the modern term for the head of the department), the professor monotonously recites the Galenic text in Latin, reading the actual dissection by an uneducated barber-surgeon whose only skill is with a knife. A demonstrator, at the right, points out the salient points of the dissection to a group of bored students, who are present only to satisfy a rule of the curriculum that several days each year be devoted to such an exercise.

More recent scholarship has led to new interpretations of the significance of the various figures in the illustration. It has been suggested that the dissector was actually a highly qualified member of the College of Surgeons and that the demonstrator was himself a professor of anatomy. It is probable (and here we have their youthfulness as good evidence) that the only students depicted are the two very interested young men standing on either side of the dissection while a group of five teachers are simply standing around, awaiting their turns to speak.

Colorplate 7. Manuscript illustration. 12 × 8¼" (30.7 × 21 cm). Photo Courtesy of the Harvey Cushing/John Hay Whitney Medical Library at Yale, New Haven.

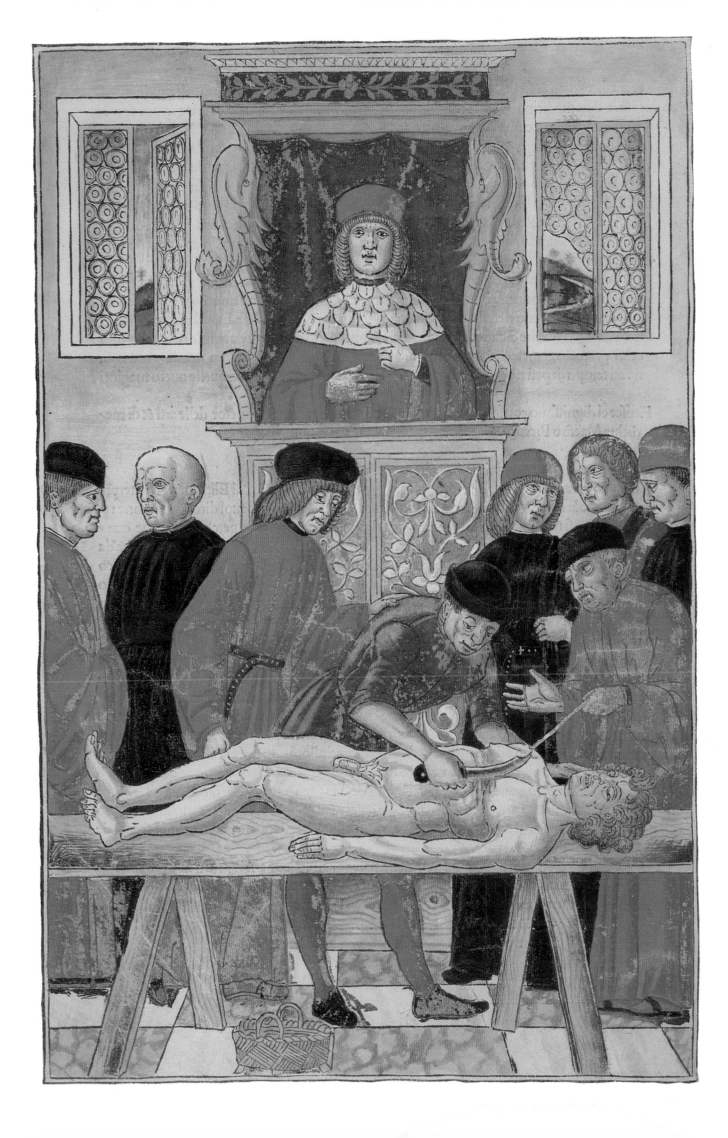

ca. 1510

Leonardo da Vinci

Although there have been artists who were anatomists and anatomists who skillfully did their own artistic illustrations, there has never been anyone whose talents at both even remotely approached the genius of Leonardo da Vinci. Moreover, there was another element that set him apart: unlike other artists, Leonardo did not draw anatomy to create beauty for others; unlike other anatomists, he did not draw anatomy to disseminate new knowledge. All his anatomical art was done in the service of his own ceaseless curiosity.

Sigmund Freud said of Leonardo that he was a man who awoke too early in the darkness while others were still asleep. Perhaps the fault lies not with the slumberers, but with the Renaissance master himself, who never made any consistent attempt to wake anyone up. His idiosyncratic script, his tendency to fill empty spaces on any available page with continuations from another part of his manuscript, as well as his own remoteness and general inattention to literate communication—these are but some of the characteristics of his anatomical work that made it generally inaccessible to scholars for centuries after his death in 1519. In his *Lives of the Painters*, Giorgio Vasari wrote of Leonardo:

> Whoever succeeds in reading these notes of Leonardo will be amazed to find how well that divine spirit has reasoned of the arts, the muscles, the nerves and veins, with the greatest diligence in all things.

By a circuitous and now untraceable route, Leonardo's anatomical drawings came to reside in the Royal Library at Windsor Castle, near London. Among the most celebrated of them is the page shown here, drawn in the red chalk he customarily used. Most prominent is the large drawing of a fetus in the uterus. To indicate that this is the first picture in the series, Leonardo has marked its text with an asterisk. His comments contain the error of denying the existence of a fetal heartbeat, but they have some interesting musings on the relation of the mother's soul to that of the fetus: "One and the same soul governs the bodies, and the same nourishes both."

There are several significant errors in the drawing, for which one can hardly blame a dissector of the late fifteenth century who still had the pre-Vesalian tendency to extrapolate from nonhuman anatomy. For example, the placenta Leonardo has drawn here is that of a cow.

In the midst of the embryology, some leftover spaces have been filled with stray thoughts. Near the right margin, a note and diagram refer to the behavior of an eccentrically weighted sphere, and in the lower right corner is a disquisition on binocular vision. Leonardo's pages are as crowded with miscellaneous ideas as was his incomparable mind.

Colorplate 8. Pen and ink. 11⅞×8⁷/₁₆" (30.2×21.4 cm). Windsor Castle Royal Library © 1991 Her Majesty Queen Elizabeth II. Berkshire, England.

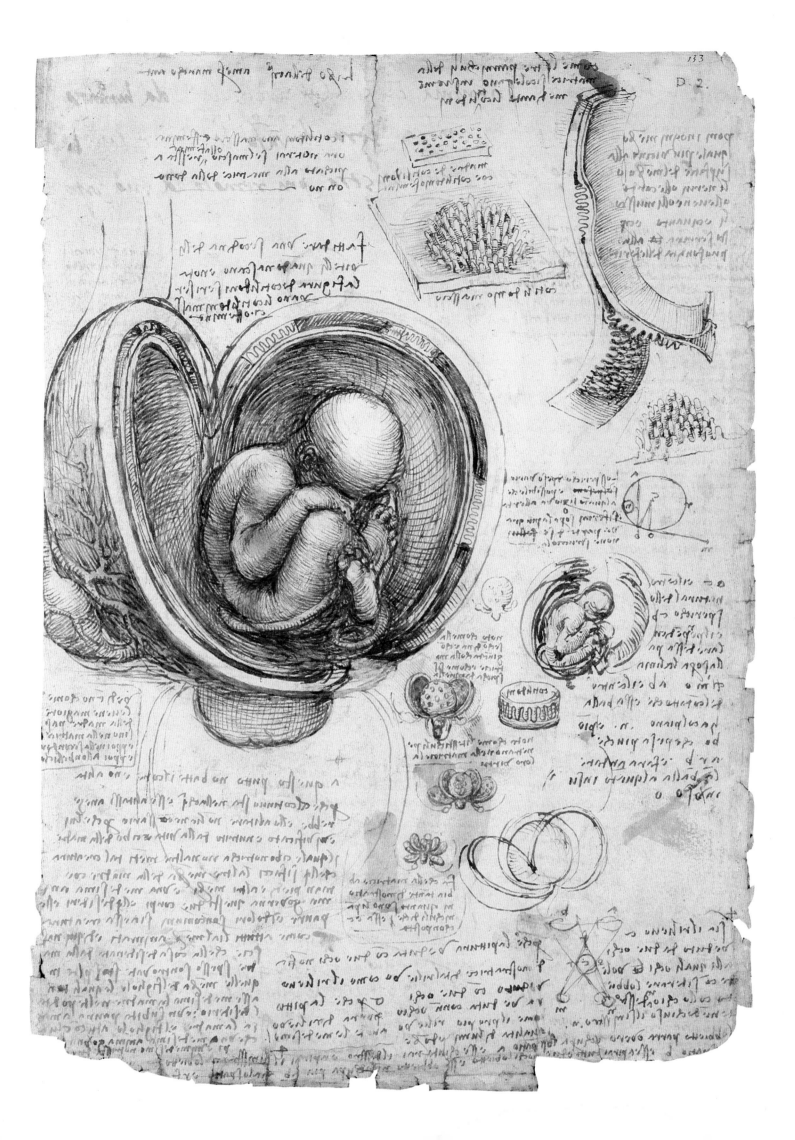

SYPHILIS

1496

Albrecht Dürer

The Italians called it the French disease, the French called it the Neapolitan disease, and it has occasionally been referred to as the Spanish, or the English, disease—no one wants to be the proprietor of syphilis. But because its first great outbreak occurred in the early sixteenth century, when the most illustrious seats of learning were the Italian universities and their medical schools, the term *morbus Gallicus* became the preferred one throughout Europe, and the French had little choice but to accept it.

The disease seems to have been unknown until the last years of the fifteenth century, and there are several conflicting theories about its site of origin and the reasons for its rapid spread. The traditional story that Christopher Columbus brought it back from the New World does not have much support among historians. The legend had its beginnings in the writings of certain Spanish authors who claimed to have seen it among sailors returning from Hispaniola. When carefully scrutinized, their evidence is questionable at best and is not confirmed by physicians' records in the cities thought to be along the routes of spread from Lisbon, where Columbus landed. Moreover, studies of pre-Columbian American skeletons do not reveal a single definite sign of syphilis.

Most likely, the disease existed in Europe in a somewhat less virulent form before Columbus returned in 1493, perhaps as one of the skin afflictions sometimes called leprosy. It seems to have changed in character at about the time of the Columbian voyages and then to have spread by the extensive movements of soldiers that occurred after this period, following the invasion of Italy by the French under Charles VIII. Churchmen spoke of it as a scourge from heaven, and astronomers attributed it to a recent confluence of Saturn and Mars, which they had interpreted as portending an epidemic of "scabies." It is this destructive skin manifestation of the second stage of syphilis that Albrecht Dürer, the greatest of the German Renaissance artists, depicted in the 1496 woodcut he made for a broadside. This is the earliest of the known artistic representations of the disease in this form, and perhaps the very first recorded indication of the secondary eruption. It presents a riddle to students of syphilis, who have no way of knowing whether the disease had changed or was simply being observed and documented more closely because it was suddenly more common.

At the time of this broadside's production, the pestilence had not acquired the name by which we now know it. That name was given to it as a result of a poem written in 1530 by the Veronese physician Gerolamo Fracastoro, *Syphilis sive morbus Gallicus*, which tells the story of a handsome young shepherd named Syphilis who had the temerity to insult Apollo. The gods punished him by the infliction of a disgusting disease with the characteristics of *morbus Gallicus*, which could only be treated by the proper use of mercury and the gum of the quaiacum tree, known at the time as the Holy Wood. Fracastoro is remembered today not only for his poetic description of syphilis and its treatment, but also for similar studies of two other epidemic diseases, typhus and bubonic plague.

Colorplate 9. Woodcut for a broadside or poster. Kupferstichkabinett Staatlich Museen Preussischer Kulturbesitz, Berlin.

LICHNICA GENESIS

1 4 8 4

Insigni Archiiatrie studio Sacrum:

Si mihi turpe putas medico cхponere vsus
Et Musis operam carminibusqᶻ dare
Nullaqᶻ Pegasei tanqᶻ sit gloria fontis
Metraqᶻ sint studiis inferiora meis
Falleris: Ille meas primus qui tradidit artes
Quicqᶻ salutiferam condidit aucto: opᶻ
Inter Pierides cythara crepitante sorores
Phebus diuino pollice ducit ebur.
Sic lustrat celos, sic clara poemata fingit
Irradiatqᶻ noue flamina docta deas:

Nurnberge Calendis Sextilibus

1496

Limb Transplantation Miracle by Saints Cosmas and Damian

ca. 1500

A Swabian master

There are numerous instances of the ways in which the two major Western faiths, Christianity and Judaism, have taken the history and mythology of pagan cultures and converted them to their uses. The holidays of Christmas, Easter, Passover, and Chanukah, for example, find their origins in the traditions of earlier peoples, as do the symbolism of the eucharist and the unleavened bread, or matzoh. Even the concept of the Sabbath predates the dawn of monotheism.

During the second and third centuries A.D., belief in the healing powers of the physician became intertwined with belief in the healing powers of holy men. To the early Christians, healing came from Jesus, and his most devout disciples were credited with great miracles in the cure of the sick. Like St. Luke, many of those who were proclaimed saints during this period had been physicians in life, but many others were simply men of God who brought their powers to bear on some illness with which they became associated, as were St. Lucia with blindness, St. Rochus and St. Sebastian with plague, St. Jacob with leprosy, and so on.

Saints Cosmas and Damian were twin brothers, born in Asia Minor in the third century. These pious Christian physicians refused to accept money for their care of the sick and were accordingly among those whom the Greeks called *hoi anargyroi*, 'the silverless ones.' During the religious persecutions of the emperor Diocletian, the saintly brothers were arrested and attempts were made to force them to denounce their religion. In spite of torture, they refused, and were beheaded by their captors.

Of all the legendary deeds attributed to the two brothers, the most renowned is the one illustrated in this painting by an unknown Swabian master around 1500. They are shown transplanting a leg from a healthy Ethiopian or Moorish donor to a Caucasian bell-tower attendant whose lower extremity had been amputated for either cancer or gangrene. Three angels are attendants. The patient is asleep, very likely from a dose of the juice of poppies or mandrake, or a combination mixed up in a soporific recipe.

Although Cosmas and Damian have been appropriated as the patron saints of several groups in the healing arts, such as surgeons and pharmacists, their legend has lately become a source of fascination to a new group of medical specialists. Not surprisingly, the modern researchers and clinicians in the field of organ transplantation look on this third-century miracle with more than passing interest. In spite of their due skepticism, they cannot resist being intrigued by the legend and its implications.

Colorplate 10. Wood-panel painting. 41¾ × 24¹³/₁₆" (106 × 63 cm). Württembergisches Landesmuseum, Stuttgart.

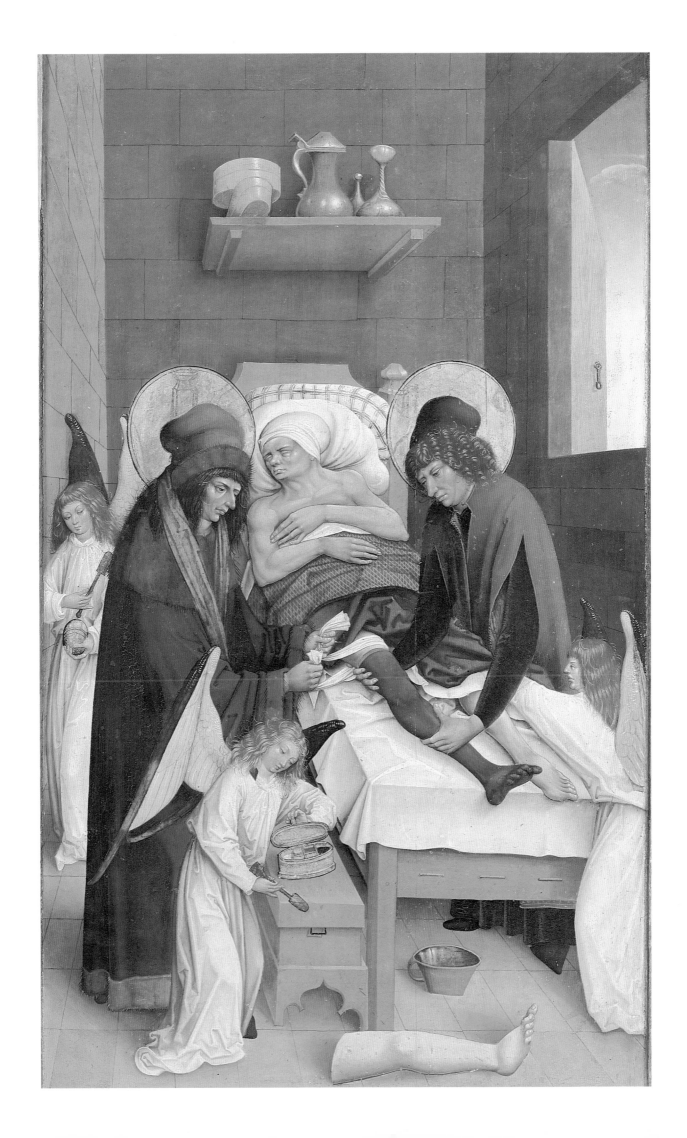

SHORT-ROBED SURGEON CATHETERIZES A PATIENT

ca. 1510

Heinrich Kullmaurer and Albrecht Meher

When a young physician of classical Greece entered his profession by reciting the Hippocratic Oath, he swore: "I will not cut persons laboring under the stone, but will leave this work to be done by such men as are practitioners of this work." There were sound reasons that the doctors who followed the precepts of Hippocrates abjured the operation of cutting into a patient's bladder to remove the large stones that were so often encountered in those days. Perhaps the most important consideration was the Hippocratic injunction which is best known in its Latin translation: *primum non nocere*, 'first, do no harm.'

Cutting for stone was probably the most dangerous undertaking that a surgical artisan might attempt, fraught with the possibilities of hemorrhage, shock, infection, intestinal perforation, and all too frequent death. Even if he survived the procedure and its immediate aftermath, a patient might still be left with a nonhealing wound through which his bladder communicated with the skin just behind the scrotum, constantly draining infected, foul-smelling urine. These were not operations with which an orthodox Hippocratic physician wished to become involved.

Those "practitioners of this work" fell into several categories, some gradually edging closer and closer to respectability as the centuries passed. At various times, and overlapping with each other, they were itinerant stone cutters, barbers, barber-surgeons, surgeons of the short robe (so-called to distinguish them from surgeons of the long robe, who had scholarly, academic training and rarely soiled their hands with operating), and finally just plain surgeons. Around the end of the nineteenth century the field of urology arose, and "this work" fell to highly skilled specialists.

In this Renaissance pen-and-ink drawing with watercolor, a surgeon of the short robe is passing a metallic tube through the patient's penis and into his bladder to relieve the obstruction so often caused by stones and gravel. Several other men impatiently await their turns to be relieved. It is probable that before many months have passed, at least one of these will return to have a large stone removed, either because he can no longer bear the pain, or because his recurrent infections are threatening his life. Although there were other causes for urinary obstruction, such as an enlarged prostate or a disease-strictured passageway, stones and gravel were the commonplace problems in sixteenth-century men and women, whose life expectancies were at least three decades shorter than they are today.

The operation itself was a horrifying spectacle. The patient's legs were spread far apart and his knees flexed backward so acutely that his feet touched his buttocks. A heavy strap held him tightly down to the table on which he was further immobilized by several brawny assistants. He may have been given a draught preoperatively from a sponge soaked in a mixture of alkaloids to promote some level of narcosis, or perhaps he was dead drunk.

When all was ready, the surgeon inserted two of his bare fingers into the patient's rectum and pressed them forward until he could feel the stone and push it toward the flesh just behind the scrotum, in the area called the perineum. An incision was made in the skin at that point, and through it a bent metal scoop was thrust into the bladder to shovel out the stone or the pieces into which it had been broken by a fine iron tool passed through the penis. If the patient was one of those lucky enough to heal his perineum, he survived and was relieved of a painful and potentialy lethal disease.

The extraction of the stone was a brutal piece of work, and no amount of sedation could prevent its agonies completely. A 1510 document says of the operation: "The cure itself is something horrible, grave, and perilous. The mind recoiled at the thought of so frightful a remedy, but what remedy seems frightful when it carries hope to people in peril of death?"

Colorplate 11. Pen and ink and watercolor. $16^{7}/_{16} \times 10^{5}/_{8}''$ (41.8 × 27 cm). Courtesy of the Trustees of the British Museum.

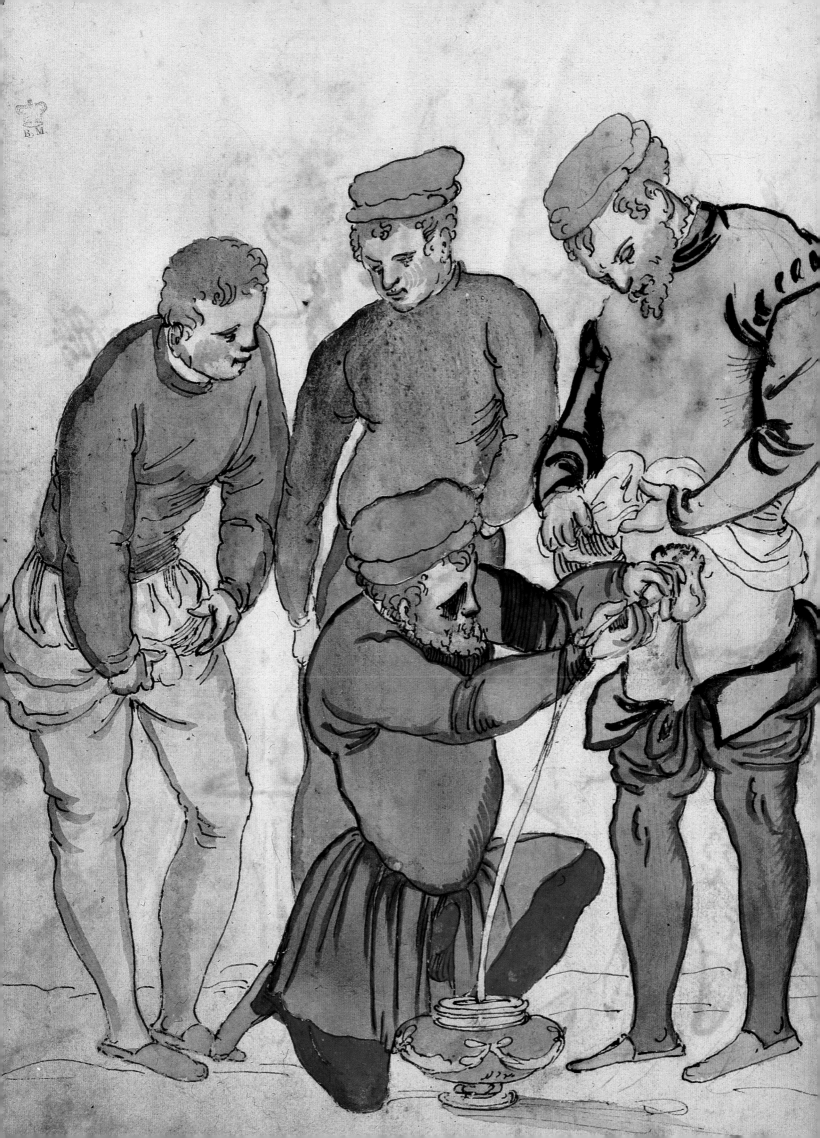

1517

Johann Wechtlin

Books published primarily for the instruction of surgeons became popular in the late fifteenth and the sixteenth centuries. Unlike formally trained physicians, surgeons did not read Latin, so it was necessary that their texts be written in the vernacular. The most well-known of such books were written in German by Hans von Gersdorff and Hieronymus Brunschwig, in French by Ambroise Paré, and in English by Peter Lowe.

Some historians believe that the practice of writing surgical treatises in familiar languages represented the beginning of a process by which the minds of European thinkers were gradually turned toward the visible, palpable realities before them, and away from the rationalistic thinking of the medieval scholastics. This trend would reach its turning point with the publication of the great anatomy based on the personal dissections of Andreas Vesalius at the University of Padua. Although written in Latin, Vesalius's *De humani corporis fabrica* (1543) was an illustrious example of the new way of observing and recording evidence.

One of the most highly regarded of the surgical texts of this period was the 1497 *Feldbuch der Wundartzney* (best translated as *Field Manual for Wound Surgeons*), by the Alsatian army surgeon Hans von Gersdorff of Strasbourg. Among the features of the book that appealed to the rough and ready surgical artisans of the time were its drawings of wounds and treatments. The illustrations were produced by woodcuts that represented some of the earliest uses of that technique in medical literature.

This woodcut was made by Johann Wechtlin for a 1517 edition of Gersdorff's volume. Using his right hand to saw off the diseased leg of his stuporous patient, the surgeon with his left hand exerts firm pressure on the major blood vessels, the femoral artery and vein. The pressure is intended to supplement the tourniquet just above the unfortunate man's knee. The stupor has been induced by an opiate derived from poppy or mandrake, or perhaps by a long drink of hard liquor.

Unlike many surgeons of the period, Gersdorff did not employ the red-hot cautery iron to stop the bleeding, but instead used a styptic of his own invention, made from alum, lime, vitriol, aloes, and nutgall. After applying the styptic, he would bandage the stump tightly in the bladder of a large animal, such as an ox or a hog. This plate is thought to be the first picture ever made of an amputation.

There are several other noteworthy features in the woodcut. The animal bladder on the stump of the observer's left forearm indicates that he is a recent amputee. The Greek letter *Tau* on his coat tells the reader that he suffered from a disease called St. Anthony's fire, which was probably erysipelas, a rapidly progressive infection caused by a streptococcus that spread ferociously through tissues in a wild, incendiary fashion. Although some historians believe that St. Anthony's fire may have been due to ergot poisoning rather than bacteria, the term persisted into the late nineteenth century and at that time was universally associated with infection.

Colorplate 12. Colored woodcut on antique laid paper. 7⅛ × 5" (20 × 12.7 cm). SmithKline Beckman Corporation Collection, Philadelphia Museum of Art, Philadelphia.

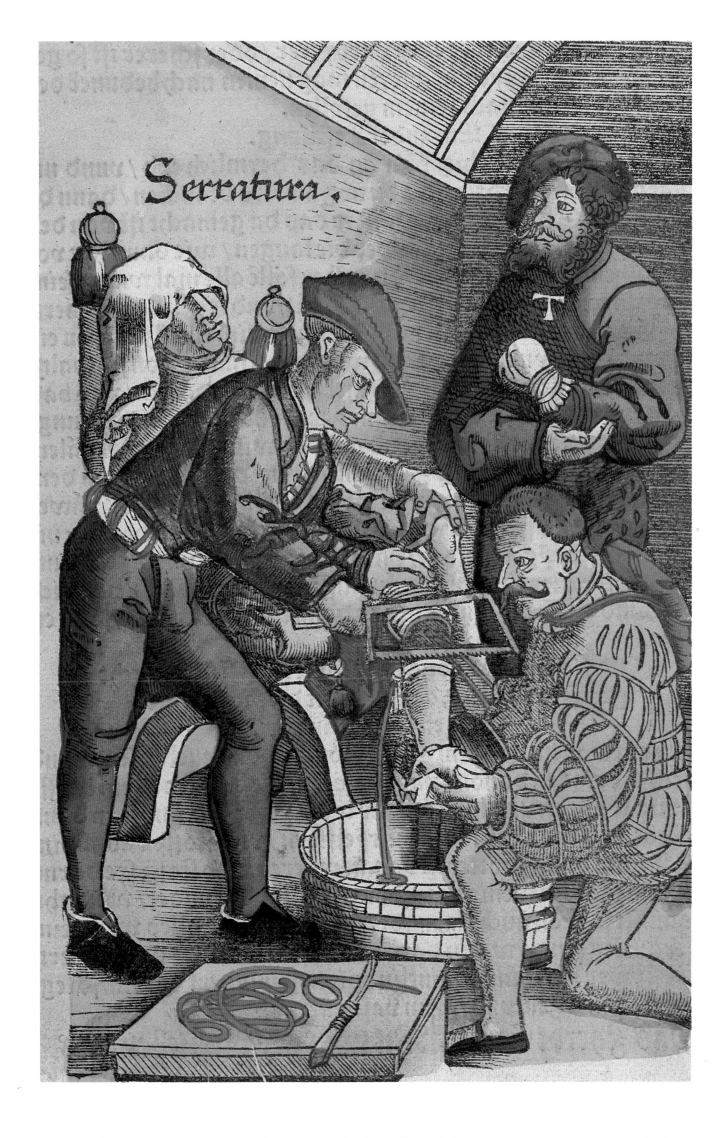

Serratura.

1517

Raphael

In *Lives of the Painters* (1550), Giorgio Vasari begins his chapter on Raphael with these words: "Heaven sometimes showers infinite riches on one sole favorite—treasures which are usually distributed over a long period of time and among many individuals. This is clearly shown in the case of Raphael Sanzio of Urbino." If Vasari considered Raphael the sole favorite of heaven, what thunderous praise is in his comments upon *The Transfiguration*: "of all his works, this is considered by all artists the most excellent, the most divine."

The medical theme of this great painting comes from Matthew 18:15, in which the supplication of a sick boy's father is translated in the Revised Standard Version as "Lord, have mercy on my son, for he is an epileptic and he suffers terribly." A man at the lower left of the painting opens a large book in which there are formulae for exorcising the devil, but several in the throng are pointing toward Christ, the source of healing. Jesus floats in a sea of light, between Moses and Elias, who come to life in the brilliance of his aura. Lying before them are the apostles Peter, James, and John. The boy is seen at the height of some type of fit that has the appearance of what modern neurologists would call a complex partial seizure.

Today we know that the great majority of complex partial seizures are triggered by stimuli that arise in a small spot in either the right or the left temporal lobe of the brain. Most commonly, that triggering spot consists of an area of scar-like tissue called gliosis. Once that focus is localized by highly complex diagnostic technology, it is possible for a neurosurgeon to remove it. More than 80 percent of patients are cured of their seizures when this is performed.

In the collection of medical works written by Hippocrates and his followers around 400 B.C., epilepsy is called "the sacred disease," but only to heap scorn on the term that charlatans used to hide their ignorance and sell magical cures. Although the Hippocratic physicians pointed out that epilepsy was not at all sacred, the concept persisted and was later strengthened by the idea of demonic possession: many came to believe that the devil had gotten into patients who convulsed in an epileptic fit. This was the thinking of many of the devout at the time when Raphael painted this picture.

The word "epilepsy" itself tends to support the belief in some supernatural cause. It comes from the Greek *epilepsis*, 'a taking hold of,' a state of being seized by some power of a mysterious nature. Control is lost, the senses are abducted, and the devil carries off the victim's humanity. No wonder that patients have flocked to quacks since the days of ancient Greece, to be treated with such remedies as tortoise blood, crocodile feces, and hippopotamus testicles.

To the profoundly religious Raphael Sanzio, there could be only one cure for epilepsy, and that would have to come from on high. It is worth remembering that the very name Raphael is Hebrew for *healer of God*, which adds a certain irony to the fact that *The Transfiguration*, a scene of divine healing, was Raphael's last painting. He died of a fever on April 6, 1520, his thirty-seventh birthday. His funeral was held at the Vatican, and *The Transfiguration* was placed at the head of his bier.

Colorplate 13. Oil on canvas. 160×110" (406×279 cm). The Vatican, Rome. Photo courtesy of Scala/Art Resource, New York.

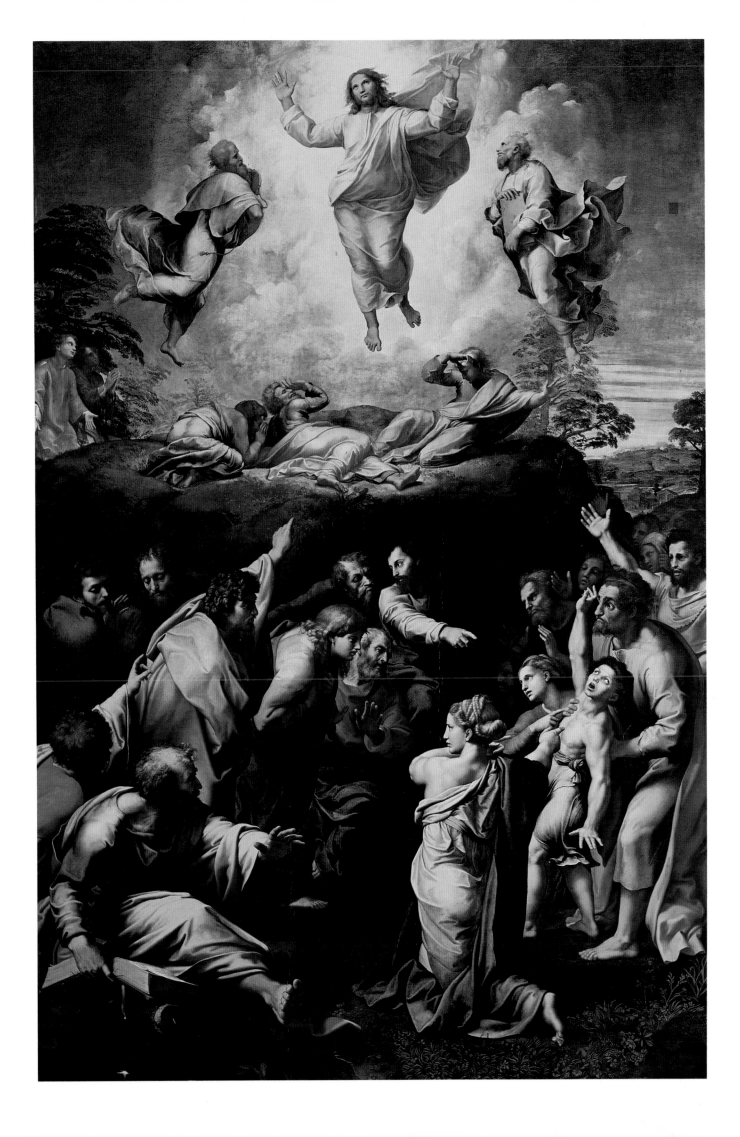

HENRY VIII IN 1540 HANDING TO THOMAS VICARY THE ACT OF UNION BETWEEN BARBERS AND SURGEONS OF LONDON

1541

Hans Holbein the Younger

Although he was born in Germany, Hans Holbein the Younger achieved his greatest renown for the work he did in England, at the court of Henry VIII. Having lived in England for two years in his midtwenties, he returned to settle there at the age of thirty-four and gradually increased his employment under various courtiers until, after five years, he officially entered Henry's service. From then until his death at forty-five during a plague epidemic, Holbein exerted a powerful influence on the fashion and style of the court. A designer of articles of clothing, ceremonial weapons, and such smaller items as bookbindings, in general he determined the royal style of Henry's period. He even designed all the monarch's state robes. In the last ten years of his life, Holbein completed some one hundred fifty portraits and scenes of members of the court.

One of those scenes is of a historic moment in British surgery. In London, prior to 1540, there were two distinct groups of surgeons who were in fierce competition over the right to supervise those who wished to practice that craft. The more elite of the two was the unincorporated Guild of Surgeons, with perhaps twoscore members who had learned their skills while serving in military campaigns. The other was the much larger group of the Barbers' Guild, who had distinguished themselves from their fraters who only practiced barbering. With 185 members, this was the largest of the livery companies in London.

The amalgamation into the new United Company of Barbers and Surgeons was advantageous to both organizations. The status of the barbers was elevated by their association with the elite surgeons and by their separation from the pure shavers and haircutters. For the surgeons, the advantage lay in the increase in total numbers and the much larger treasury of the men with whom they had been linked.

In the picture, Henry is shown handing the Act of Union to Thomas Vicary, his own Sergeant Surgeon, and the first Master of the United Company. Below the Master in rank were three wardens and a twenty-member Court of Assis-

tants, chosen from each group. Notable in the portrait is the absence of emotion or of any clue to personality on the faces of the subjects. This is a hallmark of Holbein's paintings.

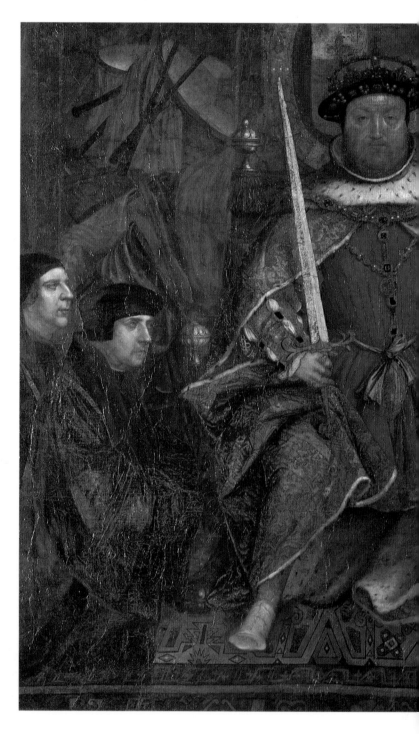

Although the United Company exerted a salubrious effect on the training and regulation of London surgeons, problems of status and income remained. Eventually the barbers outnumbered the surgeons by some twenty to one, but the latter nevertheless contributed the majority of funds to the Company's coffers. Other problems arose as well, and near the end of the seventeenth century, the surgeons began to petition for a separation, which was finally granted in 1745. Over the next half-century, great strides were made in the art and science of British surgery, which led eventually to a new charter in 1800, establishing the Royal College of Surgeons.

Colorplate 14. Oil over a cartoon on paper. 63 × 110¼" (160 × 280 cm). Reproduced by permission of the President and Council of the Royal College of Surgeons of England, London.

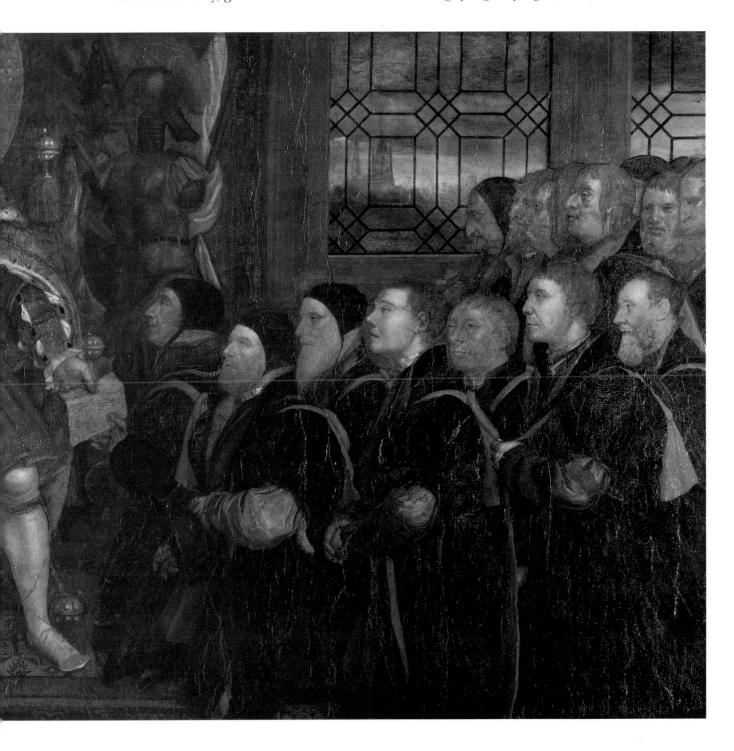

MUSCLE-MAN FROM VESALIUS, FROM *DE HUMANI CORPORIS FABRICA*

1543

Stephen van Calcar

In no branch of medicine are the doctor and the artist so dependent on each other as in the study of anatomy. And in no era of medical history have they contributed so much to each other as they did between the late fifteenth and late sixteenth centuries. It was during this century that the understanding of human bodily structure and the workings of the organs first began to be properly elucidated. This process was to work a revolution in painting and sculpture at the same time that it worked a revolution in medical thinking. We deal here with the likes of Leonardo, Michelangelo, Raphael, Titian, and Dürer.

The Renaissance in European culture was concomitant with a reawakening in the ancient art of healing. For almost fifteen hundred years, medical theory had been bogged down in the theoretical formulations based on the old and sometimes misinterpreted Hippocratic and Galenic beliefs—and worse. Worse because Galen, for all his contributions to physiology, had decreed himself to have answered all questions, and his towering authority stifled the very principles of experimentation for which he had been renowned. The earlier Hippocratic doctrine of detached observation had long since been forgotten, as medieval physicians enmired themselves in poorly translated, edited, and reedited interpretations and compilations of the writings of great classical figures.

Whatever other reasons may be found to explain medicine's reawakening, the work of one man is paramount. When the University of Padua's Professor of Anatomy, the Belgian Andreas Vesalius, realized from his own dissections that Galen's texts were based on dog and monkey anatomy, he set about to correct all of his great predecessor's errors. In collaboration with one of Titian's ablest pupils, Stephen van Calcar, the twenty-eight-year-old professor produced a volume in 1543 that would become a classic not only in the history of medicine, but in the history of education and the history of book printing as well. *De humani corporis fabrica* (*Of the Structure of the Human Body*) contained a series of Calcar's drawings based on Vesalian dissections. These became exemplary of the accuracy and beauty to be expected of subsequent works, just as the meticulously detailed text set the highest standards of scholarship.

The best-known feature of Vesalius's masterwork is the series of drawings known as the *Muscle-Men*. Each figure is shown as in motion, so that the functions of various muscles may be best appreciated. Not only does the anatomy live, but the background of each picture lives as well. When placed in proper sequence, the depictions of muscular anatomy are seen in the foreground of a continuous scene of the Euganen Hills near Padua. Modern anatomy, and therefore modern medical knowledge, begins on these pages.

Plate 15. Illustration. 15¾ × 10¾" (40 × 27.5 cm). Photo courtesy of the Harvey Cushing/John Hay Whitney Medical Library at Yale, New Haven.

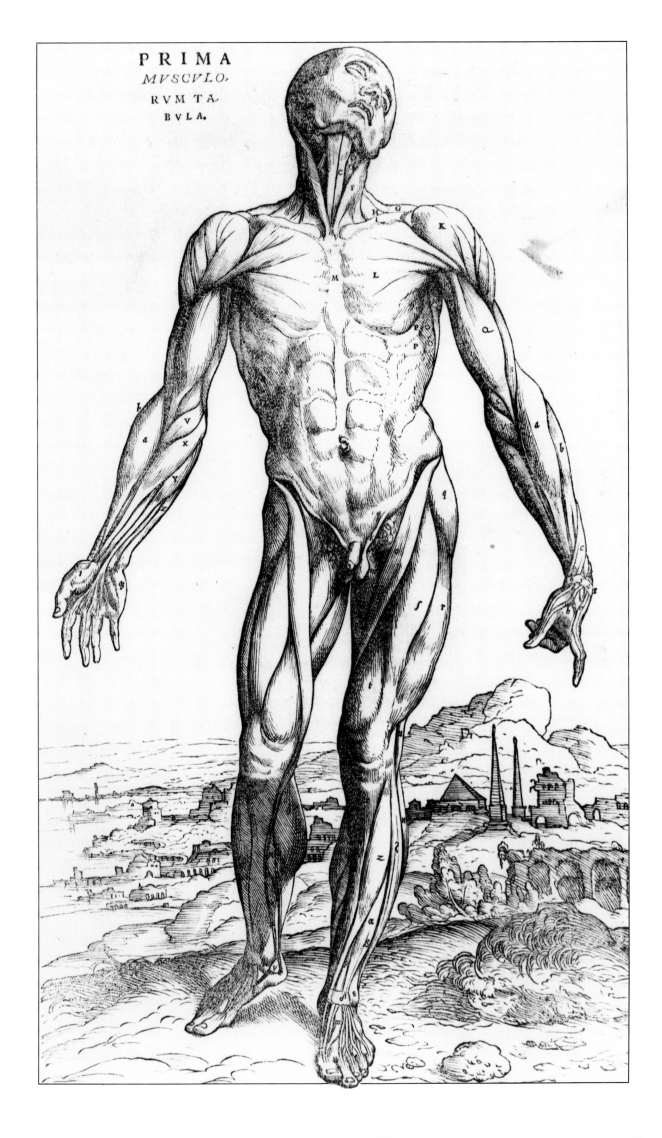

PRIMA
MVSCVLO.
RVM TA.
BVLA.

GASPARE TAGLIOCOZZI

Second half of the sixteenth century

Attributed to Tiburzio Passarotti

When Gaspare Tagliocozzi died in 1599, the city fathers of Bologna, where he was born and spent nearly all his life, commissioned a memorial statue, which they placed in their university's anatomical theater. The statue depicts the late Professor of Anatomy and Surgery holding a human nose in his hand. To those many European medical men who knew of Tagliocozzi's fame, it seemed quite natural that his statuary honor should take this form. Tagliocozzi was renowned for his successful method of reconstructing noses that had, for one reason or another, been removed from the faces of their owners.

In that day of sharp swords and sharp tempers, amputations of part or all of the olfactory appendage were not the extremely rare occurrence that they are today. Whether legal or not, punitive separation of the nose from the face was a practice also not unknown. There was more than occasional opportunity for Tagliocozzi to practice the technique he had developed. Although nasal reconstruction, or rhinoplasty, had been described in ancient Indian texts, Tagliocozzi's were the first European reports of success.

Unfortunately, the method arrived before its time and was soon discarded or forgotten. Never looked upon as anything more than a novelty, rhinoplasty was actually scorned by some churchmen who viewed it as tampering with God's work. In fact, so noisy did his ecclesiastical opponents become that Tagliocozzi's remains were eventually disinterred and reburied in unconsecrated ground. Those who would attempt reconstructive surgery were taught a lesson that they long remembered, and more than two centuries passed before such practices were resumed. In London in 1815 Joseph Carpue published *Restoring a Lost Nose* and revived the art that had been lost.

Tagliocozzi used the principle of grafting so well known to cultivators of trees. He cut a U-shaped flap of skin from the patient's upper arm, leaving its base attached to its origin to provide for a good blood supply. The flap was secured to the patient's face, and the arm immobilized by a specially constructed splint, for a pe-

riod of twelve days. After that time it was safe to cut the base of the graft from the arm and to complete the reconstruction by a series of minor operations in which the nose was modeled into a proper shape.

It was often suggested to Tagliocozzi that he take his grafted skin from some other person than the patient himself, in order to avoid the discomfort of the twelve days' immobilization in an awkward position. He knew better. Although we have no record that he ever tried it, he understood that tissue taken from one man would not grow on another. Many centuries before the discovery of the immune system, or of the body's ability to recognize foreign protein, Tagliocozzi wrote: "The singular character of the individual entirely dissuades us from attempting this work in another person." Such attempts, he warned, would be frustrated by "the force and power of individuality." He was writing, of course, about the phenomenon that transplant surgeons call rejection.

Colorplate 16. Oil on canvas. Istituto Rizzoli, Bologna.

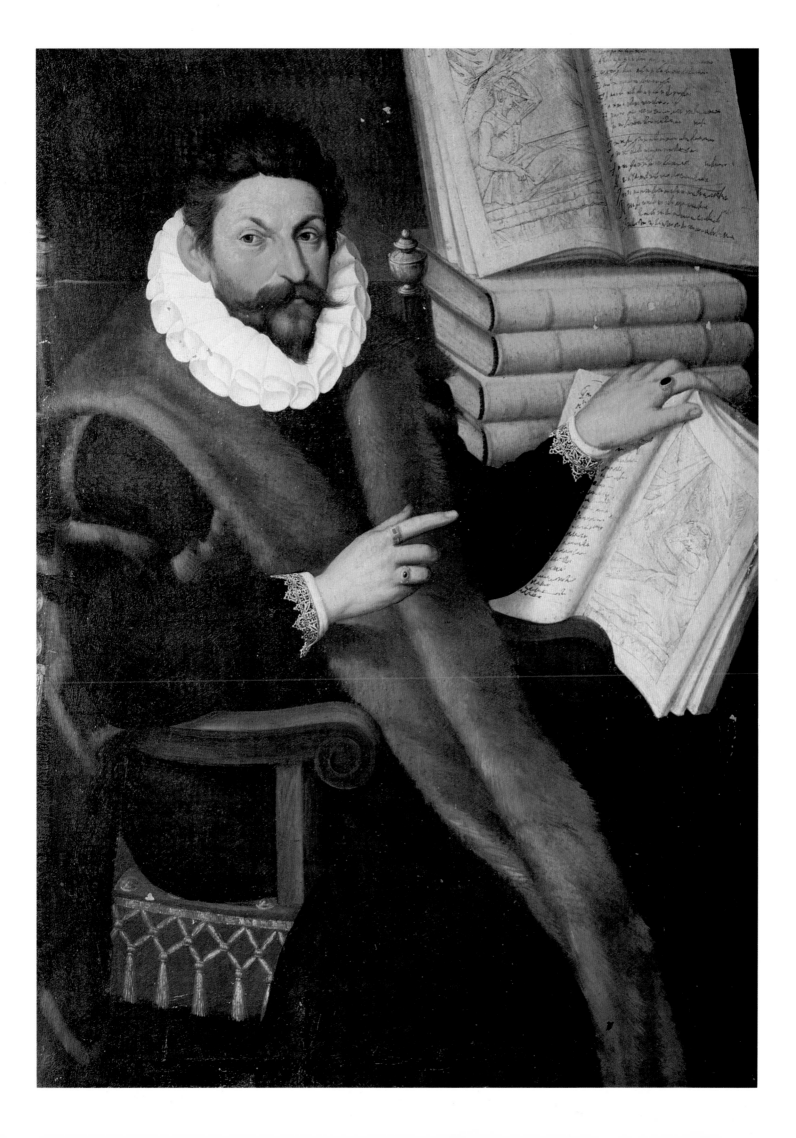

1559

Caspar Stromayr

These days, a patient with a hernia in the groin is unlikely to require hospitalization. His problem will be cured in an outpatient operating room, usually under local anesthesia. Two hours later, he will return home, virtually certain of an uneventful recovery.

It is difficult to believe that a condition treated so easily today was until barely a century ago a major challenge to the ingenuity of surgeons and a major cause of fear, and occasionally death, to its victim. Not until surgeons began to properly appreciate the complexities of groin anatomy in the nineteenth century, and then to apply that anatomy to their new understanding of wound healing, were the technical problems solved. And not until antiseptic and aseptic surgery became the standard in the 1880s did the ever-looming threat of wound infection cease to be a frequent cause of failure.

Before the modern era, many people died of the complications of hernia or from the numerous inadequate operations that were devised in often vain attempts at cure. This watercolor is from a 1559 German manuscript, *Practica Copiosa*, by the surgeon Caspar Stromayr of Lindau, Bavaria. Stromayr's book provides what is probably the most complete information we have about the surgical techniques that were used in the sixteenth century. Although Stromayr is known to have exposed the hernia by a wide incision so that he could evaluate the anatomy, his picture appears to be of a different technique, one described in 1539 in the writings of a Venetian physician named Alexander Benedetti.

In this method, the patient was prepared for operation three days in advance, when his diet was restricted to water. During the preoperative week, he was bled and purged with cathartics and enemas because "the body should first be lightened." With his left hand the surgeon grasped the scrotum so as to hold tightly the sac of the hernia while pushing the intestine up into the abdominal cavity. Using an oiled needle, he then drew a foot-long thread through the scrotal skin just alongside the testicle, leaving that vital organ free of his stitch. He then tied the two ends of the thread around an ivory or horn plate (in the picture, it appears to be a metallic bar or rod). This completed the procedure. From then on, once or twice a day, the surgeon would twist the plate held in the loop of the thread, until the entangled scrotum and its contained hernia sac gradually became strangulated and then scarred down as part of the healing process, after the involved part was lifted away or dropped off. This was a nonoperative technique, much safer than the more drastic methods of surgery, and often it was as effective. Just to show that some aspects of hernia repair remain unchanged, it was worth reporting Benedetti's comment about a "certain Spaniard" who became very adept at the procedure, "which attracted many to him, all of whom he made pay quite dearly."

Colorplate 17. Manuscript with watercolor. Ehemals Reichsstädtische Bibliothek Lindau (Bodensee).

Ob der klupen hindurch min war,
Sichstu stechen die Nadel klar,

6

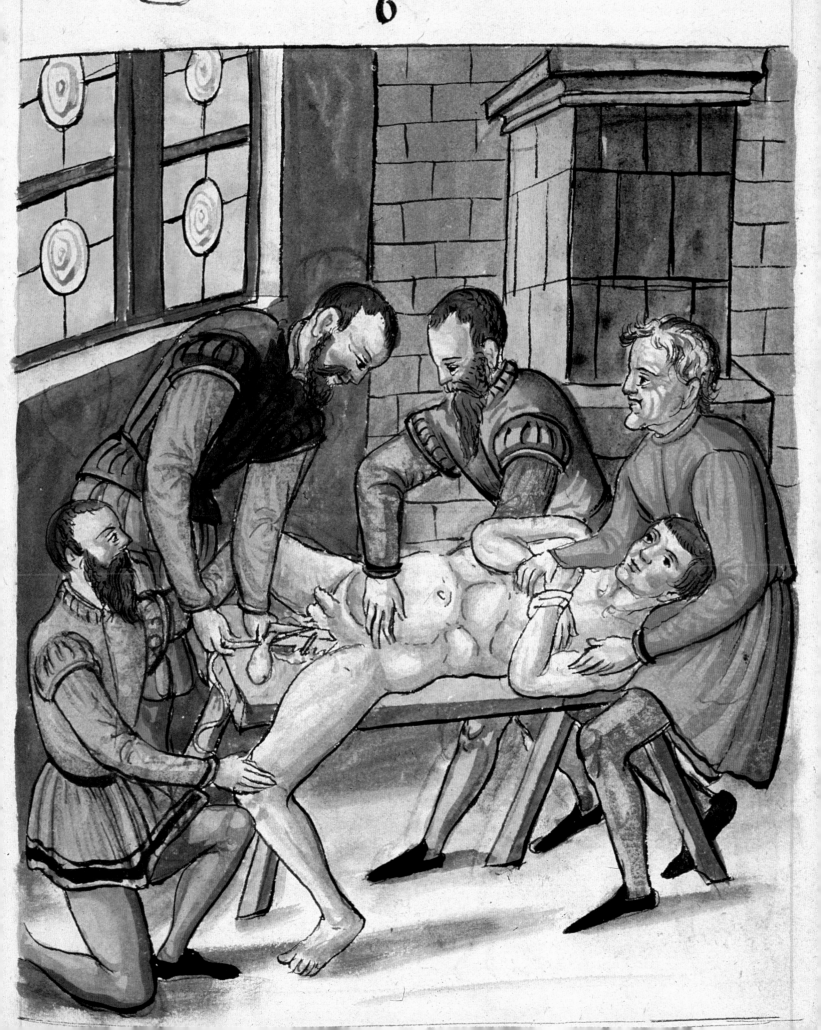

ITINERANT TOOTHPULLERS

Early seventeenth century

Theodore Rombouts Roelands

Dentistry was neither an art nor a science in the seventeenth century, and its status would probably be elevated by calling it a craft. In an age during which quacks of every description preyed on unsuspecting patients, the itinerant toothpullers were among the most egregious. They moved from town to town, often arriving on market day and setting up their questionable businesses in a convivial atmosphere of music, magicians, and jugglers. Among their paraphernalia were the likenesses on posters or banners of past satisfied customers. It was not uncommon for the least principled of these shallow frauds to claim that they could remove mythical parasites, which they called toothworms, from a patient's socket.

Although some of the extractions of the time were done by barber-surgeons, people often flocked to the self-styled specialists who in England dignified themselves with the title "Operators for the Teeth." In France, practitioners of the trade rolled the term *arracheur des dents* off their tongues; in spite of its euphonious sound, it simply means 'tooth snatcher.'

Because of their showmanship and shameless pretenses, these dental mountebanks became a common target of Dutch and Flemish painters who delighted in caricaturing uroscopists, crystal readers, and various others among the then-common mobile quacks. They are often shown in garish or exotic costumes such as turbans or fur-trimmed robes, almost always with a small crowd of onlookers or accomplices who seem to take some measure of delight in the scene they are witnessing.

The Roelands painting here is typical of the genre. The toothpullers have set up their table and are hard at work. Two of them seem to be commenting on the technique of a third who, with pliers in hand, is wrenching a tooth loose from its socket. Lying among the instruments in front of them is a powerful tool known as the pelican, so-called because its functional end resembles that bird's beak attached to a long lever-like handle. With the tooth held firmly in the

beak, the lever was pressed down in order to pull the tooth out of the mouth in one forceful effort. If the procedure did not go off perfectly, the tooth or even the jaw would crack, which is probably the reason that in Germany these rough-hewn artisans of dentistry were called *Zahnbrecher*, or 'toothbreakers.'

The era of dentist-ridicule went on for a long time. There is a famous engraving completed by

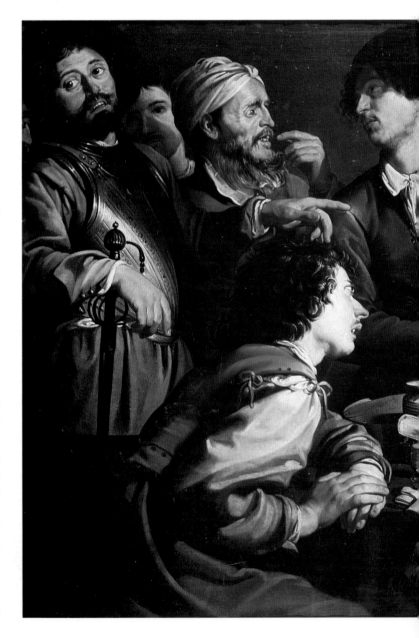

Lucas van Leyden in 1523, in which a toothpuller is shown examining a patient's mouth, while his assistant is stealing her purse. A commonly-held low opinion of dentists is expressed in the old French adage: *Mentir comme un arracheur des dents*, 'To lie like a snatcher of teeth.'

Colorplate 18. Oil on canvas, 45¾×87" (116.2×221 cm). Prado, Madrid.

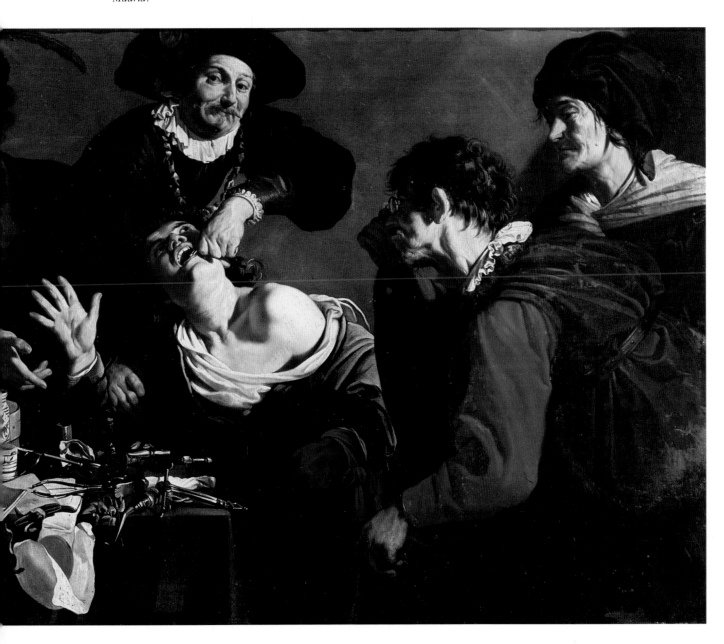

THE VILLAGE DOCTOR

Seventeenth century
David Teniers the Younger

The Flemish artist David Teniers the Younger (1610–1690) was a pupil of his less accomplished father. Married to the granddaughter of the greatest Flemish painter, Pieter Brueghel, it is not surprising that he became renowned, as was Brueghel, for his depictions of peasant life. His choice of subjects and his manner of presenting them is characteristic of seventeenth-century Dutch and Flemish art, which can remind the viewer of a candid ("caught in the act") photograph. This style has been described as resembling a film whose projectionist suddenly stopped it in midreel, showing an instantaneous glimpse of everyday life.

The moment captured in *The Village Doctor* is a glance at the life of a sick peasant, whose urine is being portentously inspected by a pompous physician with an air of gravity meant to impress the frightened patient. He is made to believe that a major, esoteric diagnostic maneuver is being carried out.

Although Galen had advised in the 2nd century A.D. that the urine be studied for clues to disease, it was not until the thirteenth century that doctors began to write tracts about it. As time went on, watercasting, or uroscopy, was invested with an endless variety of medical applications, almost none of them of any value. The urine flask became a popular symbol of the medical profession, although the uses to which its contents were put seemed to vary inversely with the honesty and formal training of the physician. Although to many unsophisticated people the inscrutable scrutinizing of a container of urine was wonderfully convincing evidence of a physician's wisdom, it was gradually revealed as charlatanry.

Honest doctors were among those who contributed to the recognition of uroscopy as fraudulent, but one of the most effective factors in its downfall was the very thing Teniers intended in his painting. The hoax of uroscopy became a favorite subject for artists who recognized the quackery involved and exposed it in very realistic paintings such as this. Particularly in the Dutch and Flemish schools, the doctor's visit is often

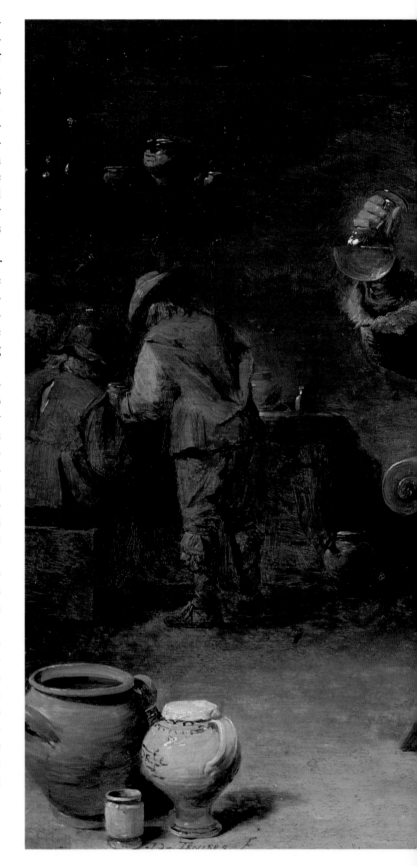

represented on canvas by his solemn examination of the urine. Not infrequently, the patient is a young woman, and sometimes her interest in her medical attendant is clearly out of proportion to any visible evidence that she is sick. Such scenes were particularly significant to seventeenth- and eighteenth-century viewers, because among the claims for watercasting was that it could determine chastity and pregnancy.

Colorplate 19. Oil on wood. 11 × 14⅝" (27.9 × 37.1 cm). Musées Royaux des Beaux-Arts de Belgique, Brussels.

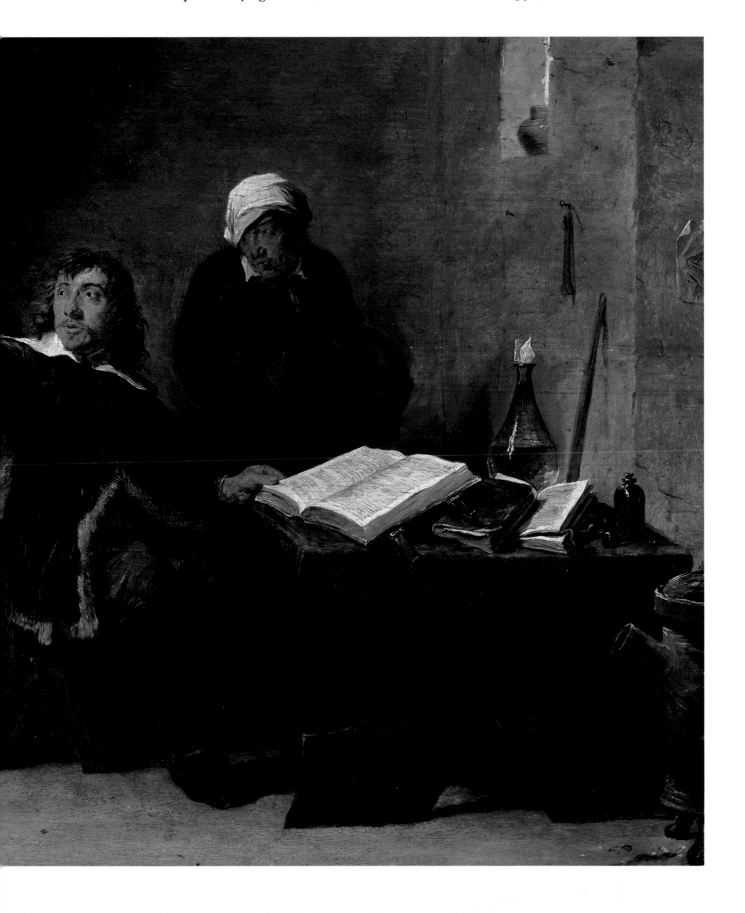

The Plague at Ashdod

1630

Nicolas Poussin

The First Book of Samuel records the fate of the Philistines after they defeated the Israelites in battle and carried off the ark of God to their city of Ashdod: "But the hand of the Lord was heavy upon them at Ashdod, and He destroyed them and smote them with emerods." No matter to which of their communities the terrified Philistines removed the ark, the vengeance of the Lord followed, "for there was a deadly destruction throughout all the city; the hand of God was very heavy there. And the men that died not were smitten with emerods; and the cry of the city went up to heaven."

Although the word "emerod" is commonly taken to mean hemorrhoid, there is no certainty about that interpretation, and experts differ. The Revised Standard Version of the Bible, for example, translates the original Hebrew as "tumors" (I Samuel 6:11, 17) and "boils" (Deuteronomy 28:27). Understood this way, the "emerods" are most consistent with the lesions of one of the two forms of plague, the bubonic (as opposed to pneumonic). In the case of this epidemic, buboes, or swollen lymph nodes in the groins and armpits, fester and ulcerate into foul, draining sores. When the biblical text refers to the "secret parts" of the Philistines, where the emerods were located, the groin is probably the site that is meant, and not the anus. Thus, it was very likely bubonic plague, or what the Europeans of the pestilential fourteenth century called the Black Death, that carried off the Philistines, whose sin was not only idolatry but failure to accept spiritual truth. If more proof were needed, it can be found in the offering which the Philistines made to God in propitiation for their sin: "Five golden emerods (read buboes) and five golden mice." In Biblical Hebrew, the same word is used for both mouse and rat.

The Black Death has been called the greatest natural catastrophe in European history, carrying off approximately a third of the population of the continent during the fourteenth century. In that superstitious and demonology-ridden period, many considered it to be a retribution for sin, while others compared it to the plague at Ashdod, yet another disaster for which the Jews were in some way responsible. A common sight of the time was the group of wandering penitents carrying crosses and flagellating themselves in atonement for their sins. But at least as common was a much more fearsome sight: ferocious bands roaming from town to town in search of Jews to stone or burn.

Although the most lethal epidemics of the Black Death took place in the fourteenth century, periodic outbreaks occurred for another two hundred years. The Great Plague of London, immortalized in Daniel Defoe's *Journal of the Plague Year* began in the spring of 1665 and lasted until the following year.

In the 1630 plague epidemic in Rome, the French painter Nicolas Poussin saw a replaying of the story of the Philistines and its resultant chaos. He was at this time near the end of his career and drawn to grave philosophical themes based on the Bible and on classical mythology. He had fought a lifelong battle with a pestilence of his own, almost certainly syphilis, and his pessimism about humanity finds expression in this example of his art.

Colorplate 20. Oil on canvas. 58¼ × 77¹⁵⁄₁₆" (148 × 198 cm). Musée du Louvre, Paris. Photo © R.M.N.

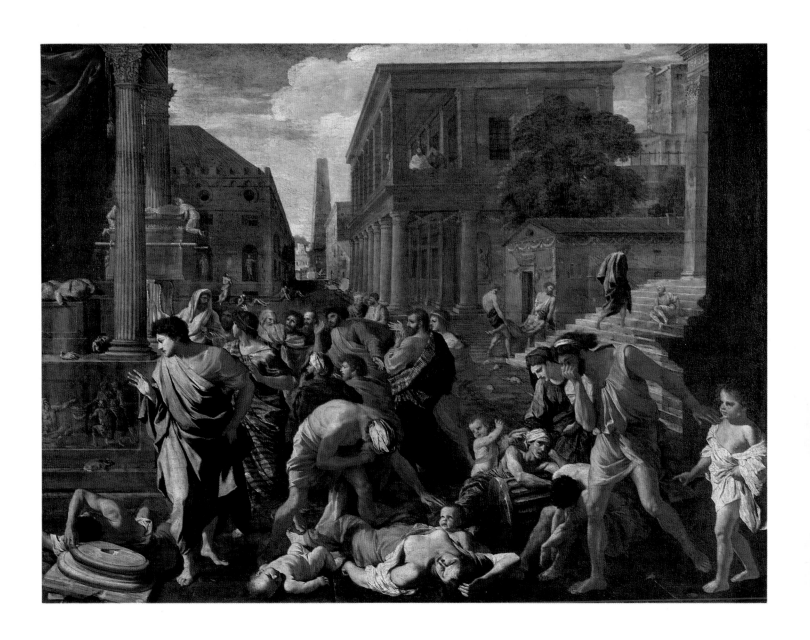

SEBASTIAN DE MORRA

Mid–seventeenth century

Diego Velázquez

From the mid–sixteenth century until the death of Francisco Goya in 1828, the major characteristic of Spanish art is its realism. Subjects are presented with such scrupulous accuracy that it is possible to make judgments not only about their physical health, but often about their state of mind as well. And yet, no matter how clinical the eye, the Spanish painter of this period preserved the dignity of each of the people portrayed. Whatever the subject's rank or deformity, he or she is never treated as an object of ridicule. There was no greater master of the realistic Spanish style than Diego Velázquez (1599–1660).

Velázquez was appointed court painter to Philip IV in 1623 and served the monarch in various official capacities during the next four decades. Some of his most interesting paintings are of members of the royal family and their entourage. During the 1630s and 1640s he produced a series of portraits of court jesters and dwarfs, of which *Sebastian de Morra* is among the best known, perhaps because it is the most forceful.

The dwarf looks directly out at the viewer, his clenched fists held in an attitude of defiance matched by the bold power of his gaze. This appearance is accentuated by the gold-trimmed red cloak that frames him against the dark background. He is a man to be dealt with.

Deformed people, particularly dwarfs, were commonly encountered in the royal courts of the sixteenth to the eighteenth centuries. Often they were highly valued companions to the royal children; Morra, for example, served the prince Baltasar Carlos from 1643 until the latter's death in 1646. Previous to that, he had been in Flanders in the household of the Cardinal Infante.

Morra's form of dwarfism, achondroplasia, is one of the more common types. It is due to an abnormality that affects only those bones that are formed in cartilage and is therefore most evident in the long bones of the arms and legs and in the base of the skull. This results in significant shortening of the extremities, with a nose that has a flattened and depressed bridge. Often the forehead appears to bulge. It is rare for achondroplastic dwarfs to grow to a height beyond about four feet eight inches. All these features have been captured by the keen scrutiny of the painter's eye. By showing de Morra with his hands balled up, Velázquez has obscured, perhaps deliberately, one of the most prominent features of achondroplasia—the near-equal length of all the fingers.

Colorplate 21. Oil on canvas. Prado, Madrid.

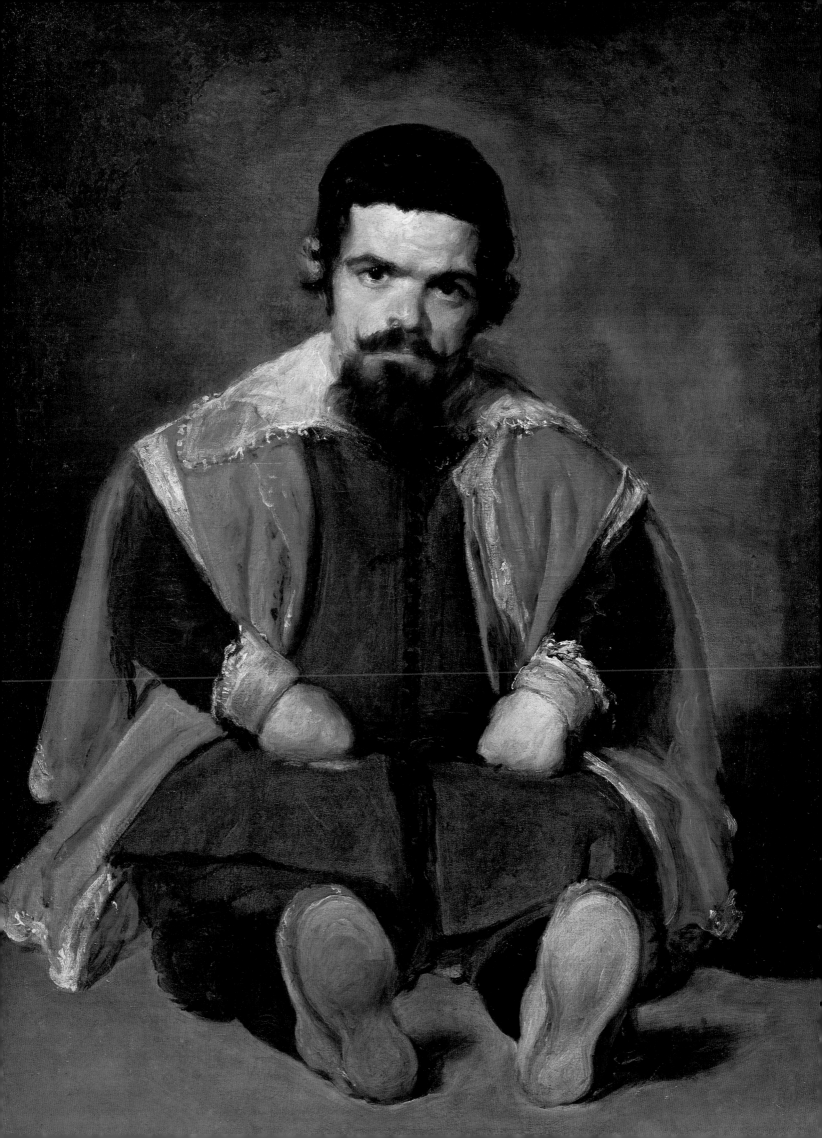

1632

Rembrandt

When the twenty-six-year-old Rembrandt van Rijn was commissioned in 1632 to paint a picture of one of the periodic demonstrations of anatomy held for the Amsterdam Company of Surgeons, he was following in the Dutch tradition of this sort of portraiture. Aert Pietersz (in 1603), Michiel and Pieter van Miereveld (in 1617), Thomas de Keyser (in 1619), and Nicolaes Eliasz (in 1625) had already produced such works, but their paintings were essentially group portraits of expressionless surgeons positioned around a corpse, staring out at the viewer. This would not be sufficient for Rembrandt or his major subject, the *praelector anatomiae*, or chief anatomical demonstrator of Amsterdam.

Although he had been invited to teach anatomy to surgeons, Dr. Nicolaes Tulp was neither an anatomist nor a surgeon. He was a leading physician of Holland whose chief interest was to identify the pathological changes that disease produces in the internal organs of the body. Autopsies to elucidate the mechanism of death were just beginning to be done in the early seventeenth century. At that time, sickness was still thought to be due to an imbalance of the four humors, but a few visionary physicians had begun to understand the need to seek further. In his 1605 book *The Advancement of Learning*, the philosopher of science Francis Bacon wrote of the necessity to do postmortem examinations of patients because "in the differences of the internal parts, are often found the causes of death." It was this new philosophy of disease that lead Tulp to a series of dissections, resulting in his 1641 opus, *Observationes medicae*, which included autopsy reports as well as drawings of pathologic organs.

In Tulp, Rembrandt was dealing not only with a prominent citizen of Amsterdam (he was an alderman and a member of the town council as well as being a distinguished physician), but also with a medical investigator who considered himself a disciple of Vesalius. The dissection that Tulp chose to demonstrate in the painting is the same one that Vesalius is shown performing in the Stephen van Calcar portrait in Vesalius's anatomy: He is dissecting the muscles and tendons that flex the fingers.

The faces of the observing surgeons are seen in a variety of expressions. One can almost guess what each of them is thinking. Although this feature is characteristic of Rembrandt's work, it is nowhere as vivid as in this early painting. Perhaps the most interesting face is that of Mathys Calkoen, who is positioned at the very center. He is leaning forward on one elbow, his gaze fixed on Tulp's left hand, which is held in precisely the flexed position that Tulp is reproducing on the cadaver by pulling on the appropriate tendons of the dissected forearm.

Colorplate 22. Oil on canvas. 66¾×85¼" (169.5×216.5 cm). Mauritshuis, The Hague.

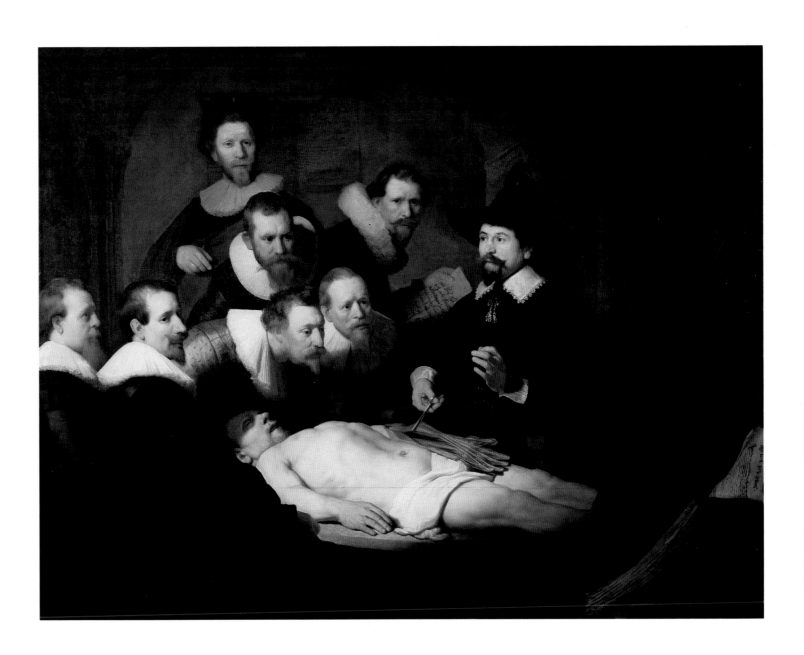

CHRIST AT THE POOL OF BETHESDA

1735–1736

William Hogarth

William Hogarth was born on a small street within one hundred yards of St. Bartholomew's Hospital in London, appropriately called Bartholomew's Close. He never forgot his boyhood home or the hospital within whose shadow he spent the early years of his life. When, as a successful artist, he was elected a governor of St. Bartholomew's in 1735, he painted two Biblical scenes to decorate the main staircase that led up to the great hall, in a style and with themes radically different from the satiric and narrative work for which he had become well known. Both of these large paintings were inspired by stories from the Gospels: *The Good Samaritan*, from Luke 10:29–37; and *The Pool of Bethesda*, from John 5:2–9. The second of the pictures is so rich in medical imagery that the viewer may wonder whether Hogarth was guided in his work by the advice of physician friends.

Bethesda, 'house of mercy,' refers to a pool (actually found to be twin pools when excavated in 1871) just north of the Temple in Jerusalem. It is here that Jesus said: "Rise, take up thy bed and walk" and immediately cured a man crippled by an unspecified infirmity for the previous thirty-eight years. It is perhaps not pure coincidence that Hogarth himself was thirty-eight years old when he painted this scene.

The angel who "went down at a certain season into the pool and troubled the water" is seen hovering above the figures. Jesus, standing near the edge of the pool, is the focus of the picture, and all of the congregated sufferers are looking to him. The cripple of the gospel story has just removed the bandages from his ulcerated leg and appears ready to take up his bed and walk.

Following a careful study of the painting in 1905, a London physician named Norman Moore described the clinical conditions he believed are represented. On the right a pale thin man clutches his swollen abdomen in obvious pain, a case of what Dr. Moore called cancer of the liver, but could just as easily be diagnosed as any of a number of abdominal diseases which a doctor would today treat surgically. Turning her face away from Jesus is a woman with patches of psoriasis on both knees and her right elbow; her maid is at her side. A woman holds a baby whose pallor, poor nutrition, and swollen joints gave Dr. Moore reason to diagnose rickets. Standing behind Jesus is a woman with a pained expression on her face,

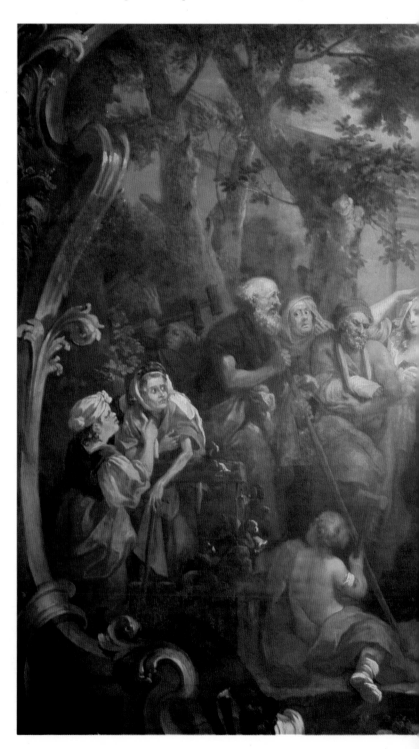

raising her arm to her head in order to demonstrate the angry redness of a breast abscess. Dr. Moore believed that the alcoholic's face belonging to the man with the bandaged hand means that he has gout, but other obvious explanations come to mind. The two female figures on the far left were said by Moore to represent two stages of tuberculosis, or consumption, as it was called in 1735. The very emaciated woman is in an advanced state of the disease, while the red-cheeked, thick-lipped woman has scrofula, or tuberculous swelling of the neck's lymph glands.

Diagnosing the diseases that artists paint is an old and ever-fascinating game for physicians, who tend to forget that in real life they would never begin treatment based on a judgment they have made with a single hard look. Until one can do a physical examination and take a history from a painted figure, we will never know with certainty the infirmities that are being cured at the pool of Bethesda.

Colorplate 23. Oil on canvas. 164×243" (416.5×617.2 cm.) St. Bartholomew's Hospital and Medical College, West Smithfield, England.

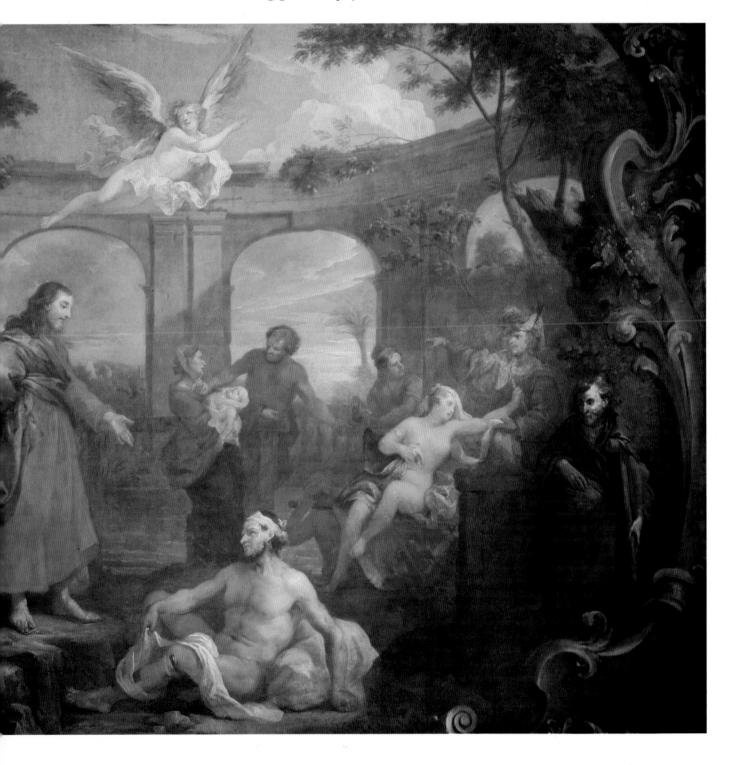

Mid–eighteenth century

Artist unknown

The date of this picture indicates that it was probably painted after the 1745 separation of the surgeons from the barbers and before the 1800 founding of the Royal College of Surgeons. The interim organization, the Company of Surgeons, trained its candidates by a combination of apprenticeships and lectures. Although the Company had its own lecturers, many of the aspiring candidates chose to take outside courses in private schools such as William Hunter's School of Anatomy and Surgery on Great Windmill Street in London.

Lectures and demonstrations were also available at the various London hospitals, where students could observe operations being done by the leading surgeons of the city. The variety of operative procedures was small because anesthesia had not yet been invented and there was still no understanding of how to prevent infection. Beyond the amputation of extremities and breasts and the incising of abscesses and hernias, there were few of what the surgeons of the time called "capital operations."

In this picture, a group of observers has gathered in the gallery to watch a struggling man undergo a midthigh amputation. (The presence of the black man is noteworthy; from time to time one of the British philanthropic societies would arrange for the training of an African so he could return home to bring the advantages of European healing to his fellow citizens.) Very likely the amputation was necessitated by an injury that healed badly, such as an open fracture that became infected. In such cases, the choice was between operation and certain death, although the procedure itself had a high mortality due to infection and delayed hemorrhage.

An attempt has been made to sedate the patient with opium or liquor, but, as always, he must be restrained by several assistants. A very tight tourniquet has been placed securely around the thigh just above the amputation site, not only to discourage the bleeding, but also because the pressure decreases the agony of the cutting and sewing, probably by compressing the major nerve trunks. It should be noted that none of the foregoing had changed since the time that Hans von Gersdorff wrote his textbook of surgery in 1497.

The surgeon is working with the usual blazing speed that was necessary during such agonies. When he has completed the single circumferential knife stroke with which he divides the muscles of the leg, he will cut the thigh bone in two with a few passes of his rough handsaw. The major blood vessels will be tied with stout thread and a red-hot iron pressed up against the raw, oozing muscle of the stump. The entire procedure will take no more than two or three minutes, although certain gifted operators could accomplish the feat in forty-five seconds or less. The final step is the application of a thick, snug bandage. If the patient is not one of the many who will die within two weeks of operation, his stump will heal in a few months into an ugly, often painful, mound that will fit poorly on a wooden leg.

An interesting detail in this picture is the sawdust on the floor under the operation site. It catches and soaks up the dripping blood. After the personnel have left the amphitheater, the jelly-like mess of coagulum will be swept up by porters.

Colorplate 24. Color on board. Reproduced by permission of the President and Council of the Royal College of Surgeons of England, London.

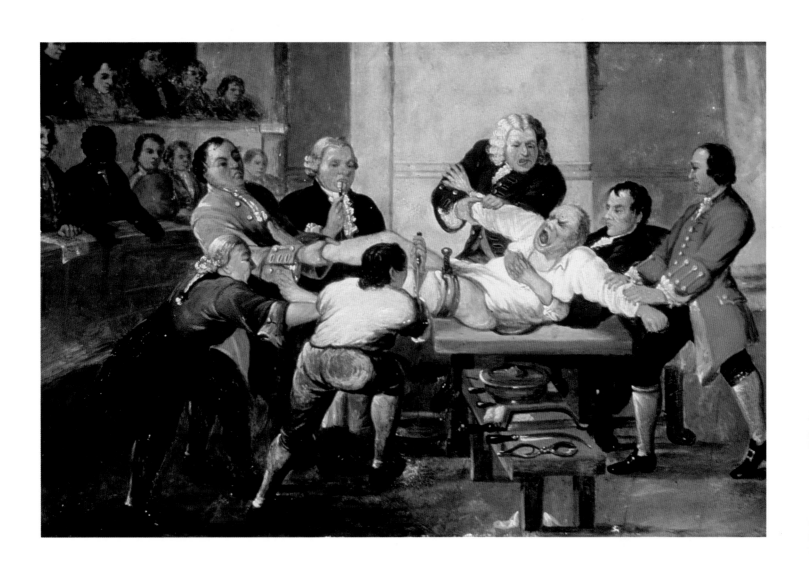

VIEW OF THE OLD SICK WARD OF ST. JOHN'S HOSPITAL, BRUGES

1778

Johannes Beerblock

When, in 1778, the curé of St. John's Hospital in Bruges asked a local artist, Johannes Beerblock, to paint a picture of the old ward, the huge sick room had been in continuous use for seven hundred years. Following the original construction in the twelfth century, three additions had been built during the next two hundred years, so that the ward in Beerblock's picture had remained basically unchanged for half a millennium. It would remain much as it was, in fact, until 1855, when new facilities were added.

We are looking down at a floor space of about five thousand square feet, with rows of open-top individual cubicles to accommodate at least one hundred fifty one-person beds. During the period when such great European hospitals as the Hôtel Dieu in Paris had at least three or four patients in every bed, each of the sick of St. John's had an accommodation that was single and separate.

By the mid–eighteenth century, Protestant hospitals were being administered by lay boards of prominent and wealthy members of the community, much like the voluntary hospitals of today. St. John's, on the other hand, was still entirely under the control of the clergy. In the ward's left aisle, the curé himself, Father Kinjedt, is seen giving extreme unction to a dying man. A small table stands behind him, on which can be seen a prayer book, a crucifix, and two burning candles. A nun is lighting a third one. Visible further up the aisle is a sheet-covered corpse being carried away on a stretcher.

While a partition separated male and female patients in some medieval hospitals, St. John's used the central aisle for this purpose, with men on the left and women on the right. The beds were made up in such a way that each person could be served from the right side. A glance at the beds in the aisles reveals that each of them has a post fore and aft, across which a rope is strung to enable the occupant to pull himself or herself up. The cubicled beds were similarly equipped.

All sorts of things are going on in the busy ward. On the left side of the center aisle, a red-coated physician is making his rounds, taking a pulse with one hand and holding a prescription book in the other. He is accompanied by a nursing sister. Further up the aisle stand two visiting church dignitaries whose rings and red coats and sashes indicate that they are bishops. With them is a richly dressed, sword-carrying gentleman and a woman who is probably the mother superior showing her guests around. The grand gesture by the taller of the bishops is no doubt a flourish to his proud description of the good works being done under his auspices. One can only hope that the tour will end with a substantial gift of money to the hospital.

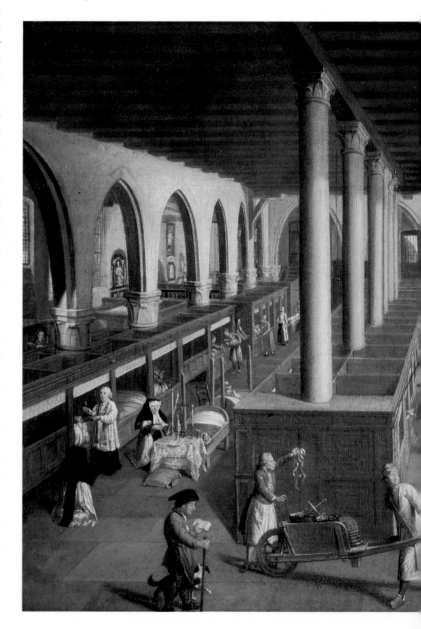

In the foreground, several well-nourished nuns are ladling food onto platters from large kettles, while the empties are carted away by a young man who has turned to flirt with the serving maid. His inattention threatens to bring him into collision with a man on his way to discard a handful of bloody bandages.

A scene of pathos unfolds at the right. A desperately sick woman has just been brought to the ward by a sedan-chair ambulance that belongs to a local parish. The nuns have dressed her in a hospital gown, leaving her own clothes to lie in a heap on the floor. Hospitals were meant for only the sick poor, because people of means could get better care at home—the mortality rate in an institution like St. John's was frighteningly high, and everyone who entered knew it. Within a few days, the new patient will very likely share the fate of the two men shown in separate stages of departing the ward and the world.

Colorplate 25. Oil on canvas. 32¼ × 60¼" (81.9 × 153 cm). Memling-museum, Bruges.

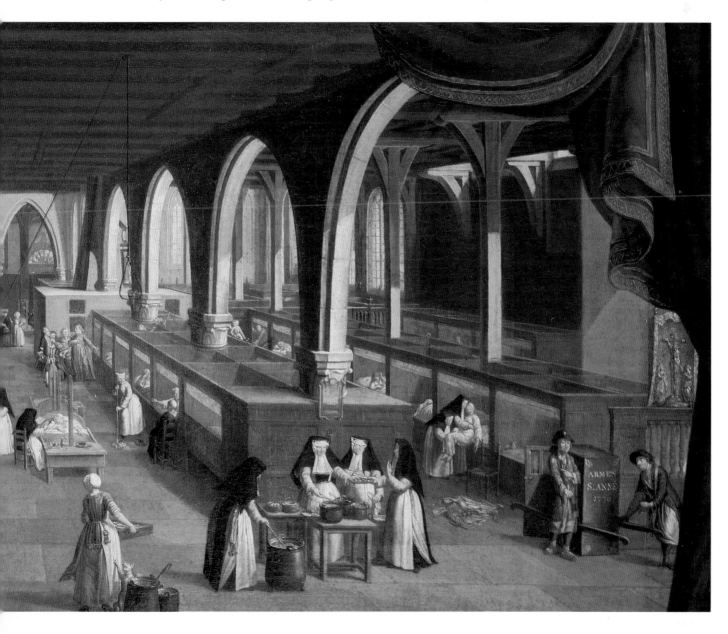

1785

J. Sowersby

The history of science does not lack for examples of Louis Pasteur's aphorism: "Where observation is concerned, chance favors only the prepared mind." No mind was ever better prepared than William Withering's, in 1775, when he was asked his opinion about the efficacy of the recipe that a local family used in the treatment of dropsy. In this condition, nowadays called edema, the tissues of the patient's body are waterlogged for any of a number of reasons; most often these are cardiac, but sometimes kidney or liver disease causes the problem.

In *An Account of the Foxglove*, the book he published in 1785 after studying the effects on 163 patients of his discovery, Withering described what happened:

> I was told that it had been long kept a secret by an old woman in Shropshire, who had sometimes made cures after more regular practitioners had failed. I was informed also that the effects produced were violent vomiting and purging; for the diuretic effects seem to have been overlooked. This medicine was composed of twenty or more different herbs; but it was not very difficult for one conversant in the subjects, to perceive, that the active herb could be no other than the Foxglove.

It is clear that the old woman thought she was curing dropsy by the vomiting and purging, an idea consistent with medical theory of the time, which was a hold over from the Galenic treatment of most diseases by puking, purging, blistering, and bleeding. Knowing that of all the twenty ingredients only foxglove produced those violent effects, Withering was led directly to the right answer. He soon discovered that he was curing his patients because the increased urinary output they exhibited was the result of the proper botanical used in properly small doses.

The plant derives its name from the fact that its blossoms resemble the fingers of a glove. In 1542 the botanist Fuchsius had formally designated it *Digitalis purpurea*, from the words *digit*, for finger, and *purpura*, for the purplish color of its leaves (although they are sometimes white).

Withering's prepared mind was the result of his background and his personal interests. His physician father, like so many of the doctors of the time, had been trained as an apothecary. After receiving his M.D. degree from the University of Edingburgh, young William settled down in a country practice in Stafford. Five years later he married one of his patients, Helena Cook, a painter of wildflowers. In 1776, his interest in botany resulted in the publication of a book—styled after the work of the botanist Carolus Linnaeus—describing the vegetables of Great Britain. And so, William Withering was the right man at the right time.

But he was cautious. Only after ten years of clinical studies did he write his book on digitalis, which was illustrated by J. Sowersby. By that time he was able to describe every side effect and every caution that must, even today, be employed in its use. This most remarkable of drugs is also a cardiac poison whose great benefits exist in close pharmacologic proximity to great dangers.

William Withering was a man with a wide circle of interesting companions. Among the closest of them was the renowned physician and biologist Erasmus Darwin, who was also a bit of a punster. As his friend of more than twenty years lay dying of tuberculosis, Darwin wrote, "The flower of British botany is Withering."

Colorplate 26. Manuscript illustration. 18¹/₈ × 11¹/₄" (46 × 28.5 cm). Photo courtesy of the Harvey Cushing/John Hay Whitney Medical Library at Yale, New Haven.

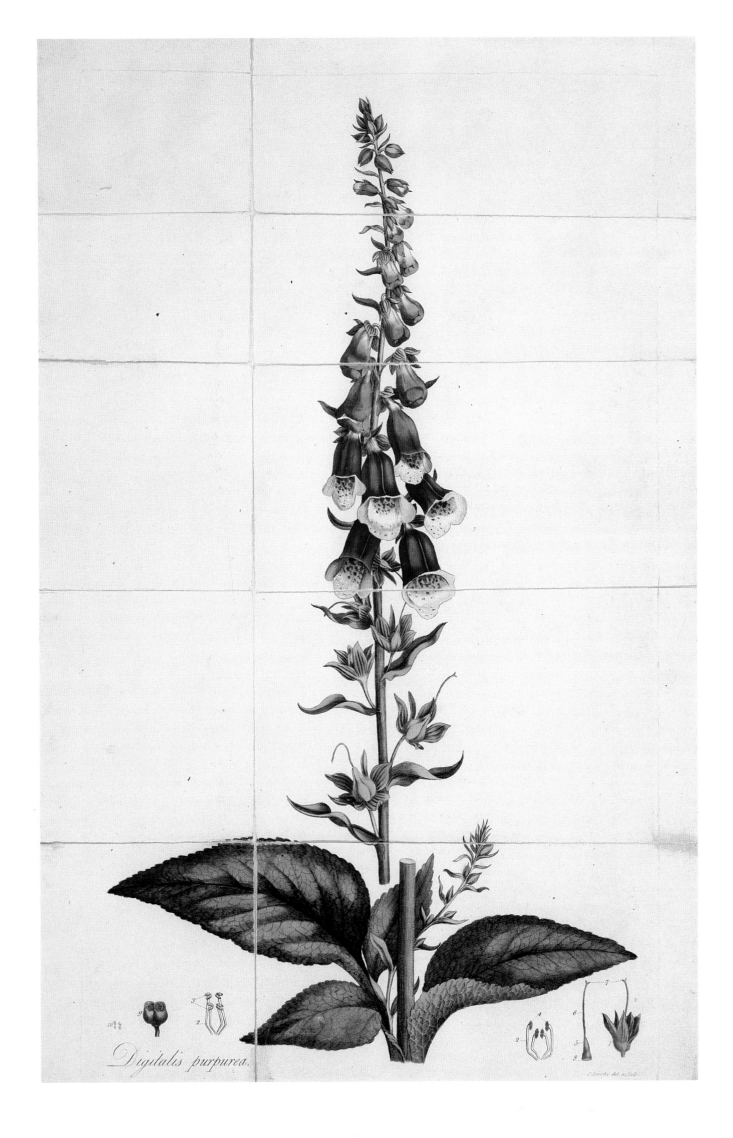

Digitalis purpurea.

John Hunter

1786

Sir Joshua Reynolds

In a time when surgery was little more than an empiric craft, John Hunter, surgeon to St. George's Hospital in London, was a scientist. It is often said of him, in fact, that he brought science into his specialty and began the process by which his successors were enabled to take their place as equals alongside the physicians. The example of his life demonstrated that surgery is a profession worthy of the best minds.

Hunter was a tireless dissector and experimenter. He believed that human structure and function can only be understood through a familiarity with the whole range of animal life. On the grounds of his Earl's Court home, in what was at that time a suburb of London, he kept a veritable menagerie of creatures, from buffalo to silkworms, in order that he might dissect them and seek clues to their biology. He was known to pay large sums of cash for his animals and for human cadavers; the story of his pursuit of the body of the eight-foot-two-inch Irish giant Charles Byrne has become one of medicine's legends.

In 1783, his collection of dissected specimens having outgrown the capacity of his grounds, Hunter moved to Leicester Square, and converted that new home into his ideal working space. A fifty-two-by-twenty-eight-foot museum was constructed with a gallery all around and a skylight roof. Every spare penny earned from his large practice was invested in his science. He even had an outbuilding in which to publish his own books and monographs.

On the opposite side of Leicester Square lived Sir Joshua Reynolds. After many refusals, Hunter finally agreed to have his portrait painted by the renowned artist. Not surprisingly, he proved to be a poor subject—too fidgety to stay still and too resentful of the time taken from his work. One day, after many unsatisfactory sittings, the subject fell into a reverie, as though lost in thought about one of the medical riddles he was constantly trying to solve. Reynolds seized the moment and began to sketch rapidly. He created a picture that was considered a masterpiece when it was exhibited the following year at the Royal Academy of the Arts.

In the portrait, Hunter, who has paused pen in hand for a moment of thought, is seen among some of the objects of his life's work. A volume of his studies of comparative anatomy stands open on the desk; the feet of Charles Byrne's skeleton hang in the background. Each year, when the Hunterian Oration of the Royal College of Surgeons is presented, the Reynolds portrait is hung facing the audience, to remind everyone present that Hunter was, as his plaque in Westminster Abbey states, "the Founder of Scientific Surgery."

Colorplate 27. Oil on canvas. 55⅛×43¾" (140×111 cm). Reproduced by permission of the President and Council of the Royal College of Surgeons of England, London.

66

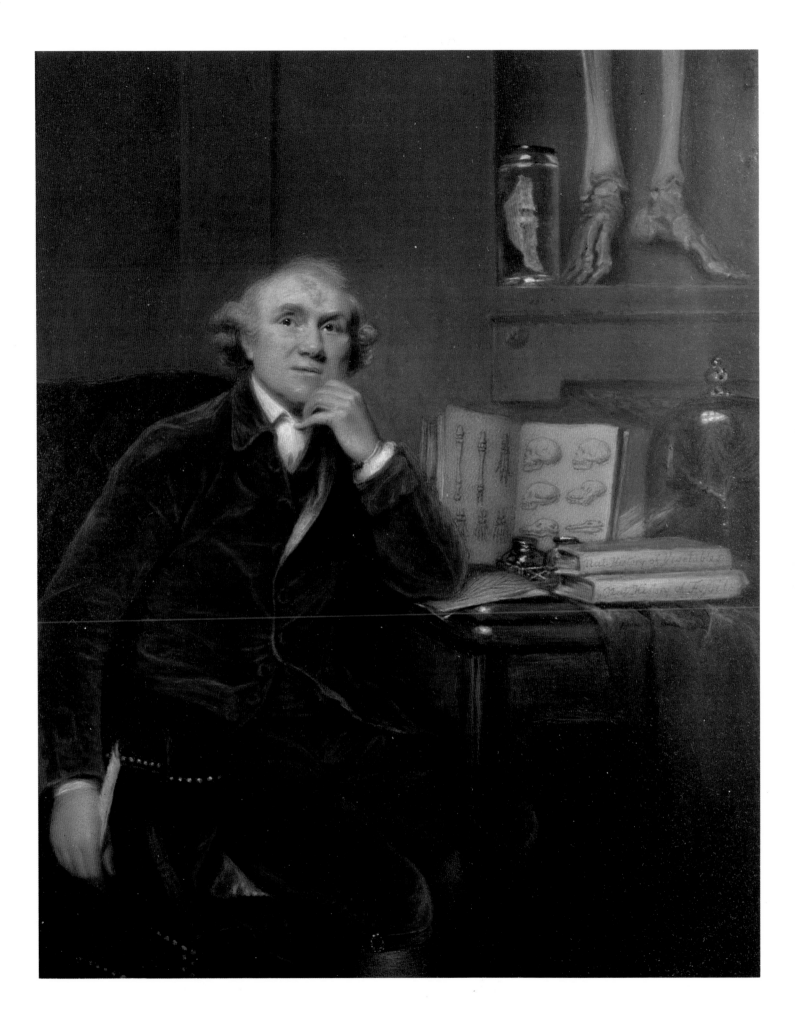

A MAN-MIDWIFE

1793

Isaac Cruikshank

The history of medicine is replete with reminders of the aphorism in Ecclesiastes that "there is no new thing under the sun." Among the very oldest things is sectarianism and the bitterness of competition. Turf wars between categories of care-givers have been going on since before the days of Hippocrates, and they will certainly exist in the future as well. The very word "care-giver" is a neologism, in fact, having been coined in some unstated agreement that there must be no hierarchy among those ministering to people in need of help. The term is a statement of neutrality, meant by those who use it to embrace every group, no matter how remote, that might be involved in the consequences of a patient's illness.

But of all the conflicts, there is none so old or so resistant to an all-encompassing solution as the one between obstetricians and midwives. In modern times, the debate was been joined in a new way; although always significant, one aspect of the problem has never been so overtly stated as it is today. The issue has become, to a great extent, a feminist one.

Midwives have existed almost as long as mankind. One of the earliest attempts to regulate them is found in a Greek injunction that they must themselves have given birth. In later centuries they were often licensed by the Church, because they were permitted to baptize newborns. We know that midwives were sometimes employed by cities in the sixteenth century, and that there were rules governing their professional work. Although physicians may have been consulted about potential problems, they rarely saw obstetrical patients or attended deliveries. In fact, in some areas, their participation seems to have been expressly forbidden. Thus we read of a Dr. Wertt of Hamburg being burned at the stake for his having dressed as a woman so that he might attend a labor in order to experience it firsthand.

It was shortly after this that physicians began to take on a greater role in the practice of obstetrics. After the invention of the first effective forceps in the early seventeenth century by Peter Chamberlen and a vast increase in the understanding of pelvic anatomy and obstetric physiology in the eighteenth century, the field became viewed as sufficiently challenging to merit the attention of physicians. The need for complex knowledge and the instrumentation that the new breed of so-called man-midwives possessed was debated at all levels of society, but a major element in the acceptance of obstetricians was the fact that members of the nobility increasingly turned to them to deliver their children.

Debates about the appropriateness of such a profession as man-midwifery were often acrimonious, as issues of morality, privacy, and even restraint of trade were brought up. One S. W. Fores, a publisher and author, took up the cudgels against the obstetricians; in 1793 he wrote a scathing indictment of their practices and motives, called *Man-Midwifery Dissected*. In this accompanying caricature, the instruments associated with obstetricians are depicted as horrifying; no less interesting is the doctor's personal supply of love potions and aphrodisiacs, seen on the lower shelf.

Colorplate 28. Hand-colored etching. 9¹⁵/₁₆ × 8" (25.2 × 20.3 cm). Clements C. Fry Collection of Medical Prints, Yale University, New Haven.

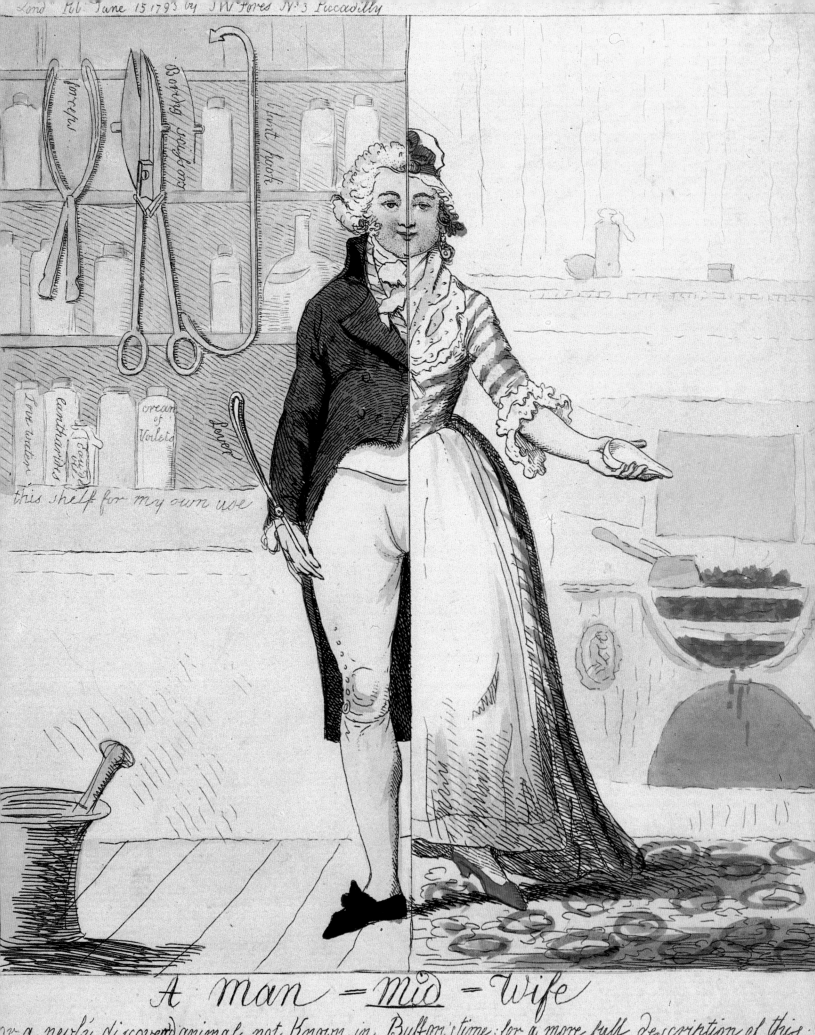

A Man = Mid = Wife

or a newly discover'd animal, not Known in Buffon's time; for a more full description of this Monster, see, an ingenious book, lately published price 3/6 entitled, Man = Midwifery dissected, containing a variety of well authenticated cases elucidating this animals Propensities to cruelty & indecency solely the publisher of this Print who has presented the Author with the Above for a Frontispiece to his Book.

GOUT

1799

James Gillray

The art of caricature began during the Renaissance. Not surprisingly, the origin of the word is Italian (*caricare*, 'to overload'). Although the pretensions and mannerisms of the medical profession were often "blown up" before that period, satirical pictorial representations began when the caricature itself came into being. Once the idea of artistic ridicule became popular, doctors, lawyers, and politicians emerged as the obvious targets.

As a rule, caricaturists have not been thought of as major artistic figures, but there are exceptions. William Hogarth, for example, rode roughshod over English society in a series of brilliant satirical paintings, including a few with a medical theme. He left no school of disciples or successful imitators, however, so he remains a unique spirit in the history of art.

Late eighteenth- and early nineteenth-century England witnessed the careers of a group of caricaturists whose works have achieved a certain trenchant immortality. The most prominent of them were James Gillray, Thomas Rowlandson, and Isaac and George Cruikshank. Gillray, although his darts were aimed primarily at the political and social foibles of his generation, produced some works that are vividly accurate in their cartooning of medical subjects.

Gillray, born in 1775, was apprenticed to a letter engraver, but he ran away to join a company of strolling players. He produced his first caricature when he was twenty-two, and he did not stop until he fell victim to insanity at the age of fifty-four. During the intervening years, he engraved nearly twelve hundred of his remarkable drawings, which he did in the form of broadsheets.

The meaning of most caricatures is multiple. Overtly drawn to ridicule and heckle, they also serve to make an authoritarian figure less threatening. For this reason, not only the doctor but also the disease, could be the foe. Until long after the time of Gillray, disease was thought to be mysterious; against its secret forces humankind fought with indifferent results. No one knew what caused it, and, in spite of claims to the contrary, doctors did not frequently cure it. By making fun of its horrors, potential victims allowed themselves some sense of power.

In Gillray's day, the disease most frequently cartooned was gout. Not only does its arthritis produce a particularly agonizing form of pain, but it was known to occur primarily among obese, sedentary upper-class members who ate and drank too much. Even better, it was a great source of income for physicians with wealthy clientele. An anonymous caricature of the time illustrates a doctor thanking his patient's chef because, as he says in the word-balloon, his "ingenious art of poisoning enables us medical men to ride in our carriages; without your assistance we should all go on foot."

Colorplate 29. Coloured and soft-ground etching. 10¹/₁₆ × 14¹/₁₆" (25.5 × 35.7 cm). Philadelphia Museum of Art, Philadelphia. Purchased: SmithKline Beckman Corporation.

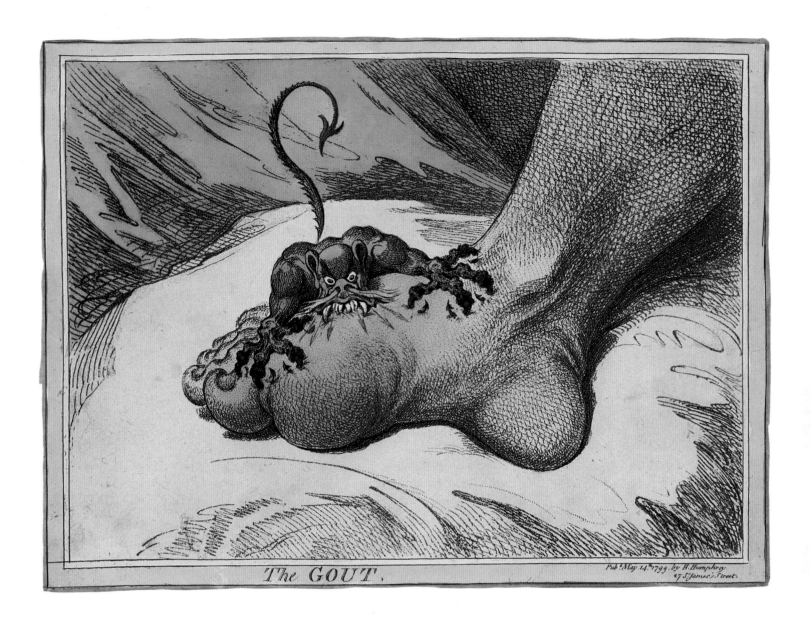

The GOUT.

Pub.d May 14.th 1799. by H. Humphry
27 S.t James's Street.

GEORGE WASHINGTON IN HIS LAST ILLNESS, ATTENDED BY DOCTORS CRAIK AND BROWN

ca. 1800

Friday, December 13, 1799, was an unlucky date for George Washington and for the young nation he had so recently led into existence. Having been severely exposed on the previous day to "rain, hail, and snow falling alternately, with a cold wind," he began to complain on that morning of a sore throat, which by the evening had developed into an increasing hoarseness. At 3:00 A.M., Washington awakened his wife Martha, saying that he felt sick and feverish. Scarcely twenty hours later, he was dead. The cause of his unexpected demise has been debated for almost two hundred years.

The most reliable information about Washington's last hours comes from a statement published by the *Times* of Alexandria, Virginia, on December 19, by two of his physicians, James Craik and Elisha Dick. The third doctor in attendance, Gustavus Brown, had by then returned to his home in Port Tobacco and was therefore unavailable to add his signature.

According to the account in the *Times*, the diagnosis was *cynanche trachealis*, a catch-all term to which an entire chapter was devoted in a textbook written in 1781 by William Cullen, one of the most respected authorities of the time and a professor at the medical school of the University of Edinburgh, from which Doctors Craik and Dick had graduated. *Cynanche trachealis*, which Cullen equated with quinsy, referred to any of a variety of upper airway inflammations that have come to be separated into such ailments as croup, tonsillitis, diphtheria, and others.

Before any of the doctors arrived, their patient had been bled by one of his plantation overseers, of some twelve to fourteen ounces, at his own request. He had then further endured what are described as "two copious bleedings" during the afternoon, followed by another of thirty-two ounces. He was also given a strong laxative and had "a copious discharge from the bowels." Even assuming that each of the two unspecified bloodlettings was no more than the fourteen ounces taken at Washington's bidding by the overseer (although each might have been more than twice

that amount), the total is the equivalent of a 4½-pint hemorrhage over a period of no more than twenty hours, plus the amount of fluid that might have been lost as a result of the cathartic. If Washington died as his physicians describe it ("retaining the full possession of his intellect, he expired without a struggle"), it must be seriously considered that he was bled and purged until his blood and fluid volume was too low to sustain life.

Heroic bleeding, as some historians call it, was consistent with contemporary theories about the treatment of inflammation, loosely based as they still were on the old Greek concepts of humoral imbalance. Dr. Dick, in fact, was a graduate of the University of Pennsylvania, where he had come under the influence of the famous Dr. Benjamin Rush, a leading exponent of large-scale exsanguination. The three doctors who treated Washington were universally considered to be very competent and well trained for their time; as recently as the Revolutionary War, only one hundred of the twelve hundred physicians in the Colonial Army had a medical school degree.

If, on the other hand, the revered Washington died in a great deal more distress, and perhaps in strangulating agony, than his physicians were willing to describe to their grieving fellow-citizens, it is necessary to quickly diagnose a disease of such wildfire progression that it can kill within less than thirty-six hours from the onset of its most minimal symptoms. Washington's pain, hoarseness, inability to swallow, and lightning decline all fit the description of a condition, identified relatively recently, called acute epiglottitis, caused by an infection with the bacterium *Haemophilas influenzae* type b. Perhaps this was the disease, abetted by the shock resulting from a profound decrease in circulating blood volume, that took the life of George Washington.

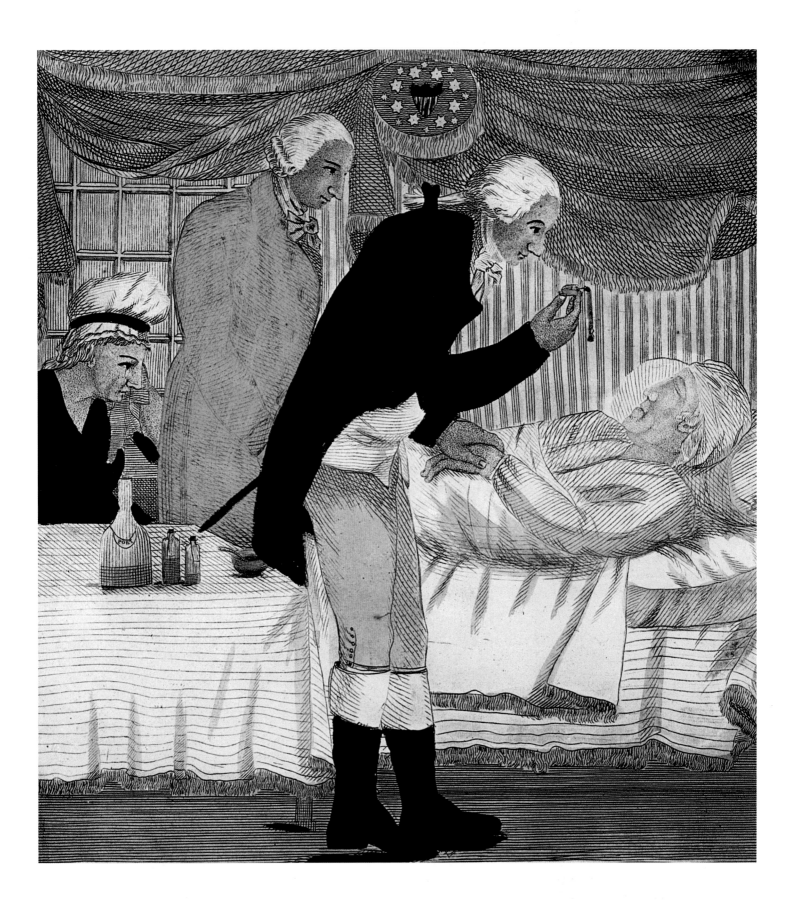

DIPHTHERIA

1802–1812

Francisco Goya

The realism in the works of Francisco Goya was inspired by two sources, Velázquez and Nature herself. Goya's son said of him that he "looked with veneration at Velázquez and Rembrandt, but above all he studied and looked at Nature, whom he called his mistress." In this, he resembles the physicians of his time, who, as William Harvey had taught, would understand nothing of their art unless they looked to Nature as their guide.

Perhaps Goya's deafness, which developed in 1792 following an illness, shaped his visual perception of the world and taught him that realism can be made even more real with a bit of exaggeration, or at least some sense of extravagance. In *Diphtheria*, he shows us a vivid portrait of one of the most lethal of childhood diseases, diphtheria. The physician holds his patient immobile with a firm grip on the neck, while the fingers of his other hand probe deeply into the boy's mouth.

At the time this painting was made, in the first decade of the nineteenth century, "croup" was the name still given by many doctors to any of several diseases characterized by an extensive inflammation of the throat and an obstruction of the upper airway so severe that it often amounted to strangulation. It was for this reason that the Spanish called it *El Garrotillo*, which is the original title of this painting.

Actually, knowledgeable physicians of the time were aware that most croup had already been recognized about twenty-five years earlier by a New York physician, Richard Bayley, as falling into one of two categories. Performing autopsies on two young children who died of that disease, Bayley noted that it was possible to distinguish between what was called *angina trachealis*, or 'putrid sore throat,' on the one hand, and membranous croup on the other. *Angina trachealis*, which is ulcerated and foul-smelling, is a treacherous, very advanced version of streptococcal sore throat. Membranous croup is diphtheria.

The major pathology in diphtheria is the presence of a tenacious white membrane that lines the airway and gradually chokes the helpless child to death. In the time of Goya, the only effective treatment for advanced cases was to reach into the patient's throat with fingers or forceps in an attempt to tear the membrane free and relieve the obstruction. Although it appears that the physician in Goya's painting is examining the child, he is very likely about to plunge his fingers down the boy's throat, and that is precisely why he is holding him in such a firm grip.

Colorplate 31. Oil on canvas. 31½ × 25⅝" (80 × 65 cm). Doña Carmen Marañon, Viuda de Fernández de Araoz, Madrid.

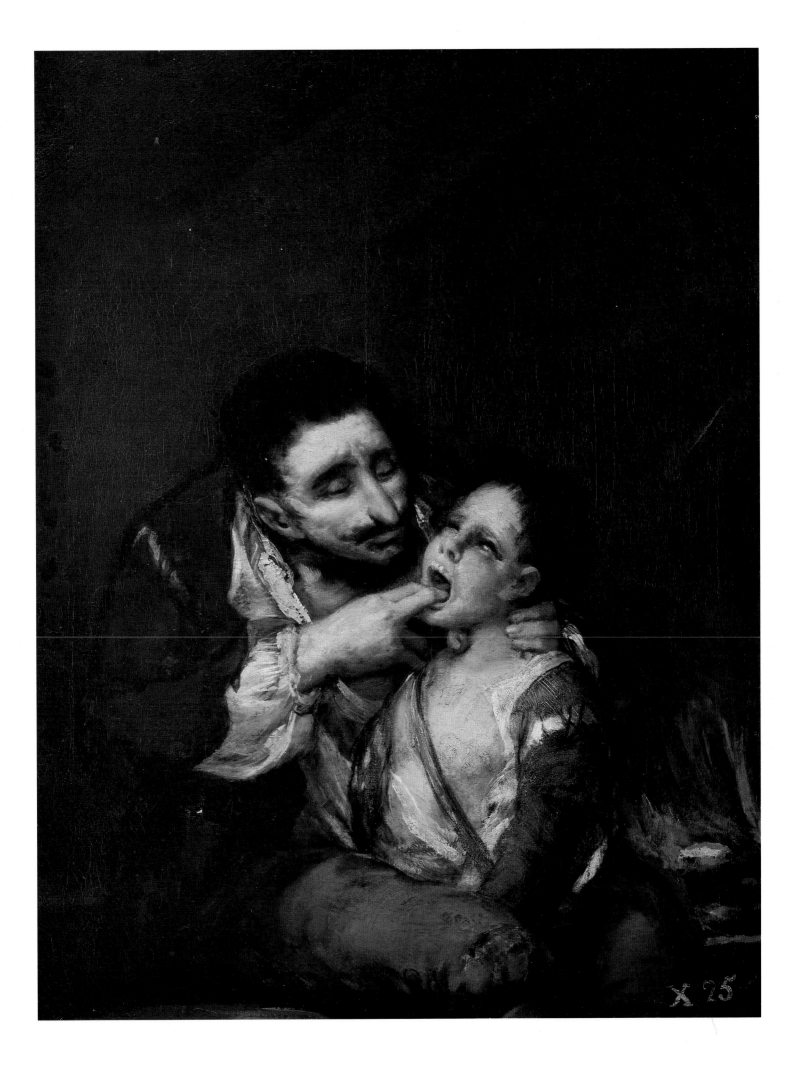

THE ANATOMIST

Early nineteenth century

Thomas Rowlandson

Of all the medical caricaturists, Thomas Rowlandson was the most prolific and is the best-known today. Although he began his artistic career as a very successful painter of oils and watercolors, he is most remembered for his thirteen hundred satirical prints, of which fifty deal with medical themes. He learned about anatomy and anatomists at the Royal Academy of Art, from no less distinguished a figure than Dr. William Hunter, brother of the renowned John and an eminent medical authority in his own right.

Rowlandson illustrated the works of Oliver Goldsmith, the physician, and Tobias Smollett, the surgeon, as well as those of two writers known for their humorous digs at doctors, Laurence Sterne and Henry Fielding. His frequent supper companion was Dr. John Wolcot, a lapsed physician who wrote satiric verse. Indeed, Rowlandson steeped his life in doctors.

Rowlandson lived at a time when cultured people still believed it possible to learn everything that was known to mankind. The anatomic demonstrations of such lecturers as William Hunter in London and Robert Knox in Edinburgh attracted all manner of intelligentsia, and even became attractions for tourists. It was an open secret that many of the corpses dissected by these anatomists had been obtained by questionable means.

Cadavers were less difficult to acquire in Catholic countries than elsewhere. Papal decisions during the Renaissance had allowed for the needs of the universities and artists, but no such arrangements existed in Protestant countries. In England, Scotland, and the United States, a flourishing trade was developed by a singular group of entrepreneurs who ransacked the fresh graves of the newly dead and sold their contents to surgeons and anatomists. Because they raised the dead, the new artisans were called Resurrectionists when conversation was meant to be witty, but a more familiar sobriquet was "sack-em-up men." This term derived from the method used to package the goods during transportation from grave to dissecting room. To avoid involvement and the appearance of implication, the customer rarely dealt with the graverobbers directly, the actual purchase being carried out by an employee. In that way, the medical man could claim that he had no idea of the means by which the specimen had been acquired.

In Rowlandson's *The Anatomist*, the doctor is preparing his grisly instruments, trying to ignore the desperate importuning of the young woman that he desist from his plans. A man has smuggled his way into the house in a Resurrectionist's sack, no doubt intent on a tryst with the buxom lass, but the anatomist has arrived earlier than expected and is intent on setting about his work. We can only guess whether the frightened woman is the doctor's daughter or his young wife.

Colorplate 32. Colored etching. 13¾ × 9⅝" (35 × 24.5 cm). Photo courtesy of the C. C. Fry Collection of Medical Prints, Yale University, New Haven.

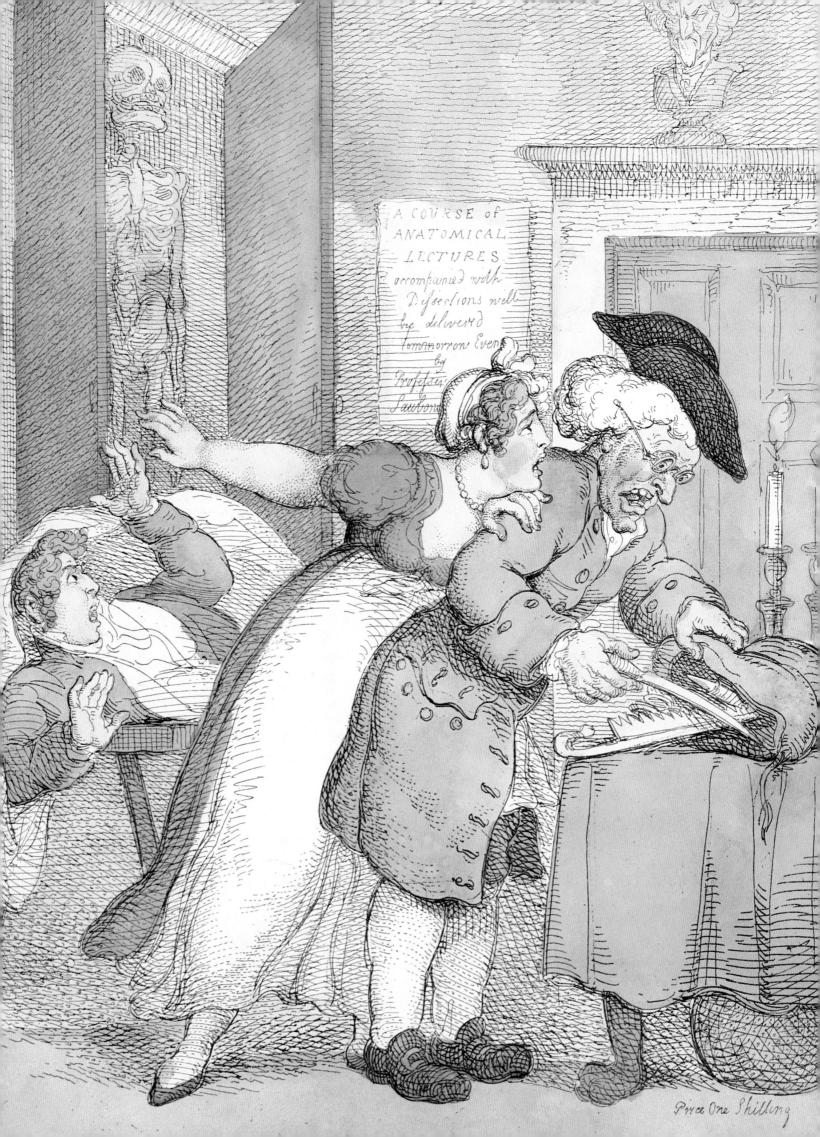

A COURSE of ANATOMICAL LECTURES accompanied with Dissections will be delivered Tomorrow Evening by Professor Saubon

Price One Shilling

SHOWING THE RESULTS OF A CATARACT OPERATION AT THE HÔTEL DIEU, PARIS

Nineteenth century

Artist unknown

Following the French Revolution in 1789, the old medical colleges were closed, and a new system for educating doctors was instituted. The focus of teaching was the hospital itself; direct observation of patients, both the living and the dead, was the outstanding feature of the curriculum. No longer determined by personal connections, professorships in the new system were granted strictly on the principle of *egalité*, in the form of public competition by the most qualified candidates.

The result of the arrangement was nothing short of miraculous. By the early years of the nineteenth century, the old guard of entrenched incompetents had been replaced by a group of brilliant and relatively young men who were making rapid progress in the diagnosis and treatment of disease. They taught not by boring lecture but by example at the bedside, in the operating theater, and in the autopsy room. At least once daily, each professor and a retinue of students made meticulous rounds on the wards, scrutinizing the physical findings of their patients and dissecting their corpses when they died, in order to correlate signs and symptoms with the underlying organ disturbances that caused them. In this way, the principles of the modern physical examination were developed—and the modern autopsy as well. The great Paris teaching hospitals became magnets that attracted young physicians from America and all of Europe.

The most prominent French surgeon of the time was the imperious Guillaume Dupuytren, who had risen from humble circumstances to become *Chirurgien en Chef* at the Hôtel Dieu, a huge hospital of some fourteen hundred beds on the Ile de la Cité. His daily rounds began promptly at 6:00 A.M., and they lasted three hours, during which the dictatorial professor taught his followers by harshness and often by ridicule. The students and even the visitors accepted his demeaning ways, not only because they had no choice, but also because in all of Europe there was no surgeon who understood the mysteries of pathology and its treatment better than their acerbic teacher.

Dupuytren was even more unkind to the helpless patients on his wards than he was to those young men who had come to him to learn. It was not unknown for him to strike a sick man. Worse, one of his habits was to grasp a patient's nose, as though it were a handle, and then pull him down

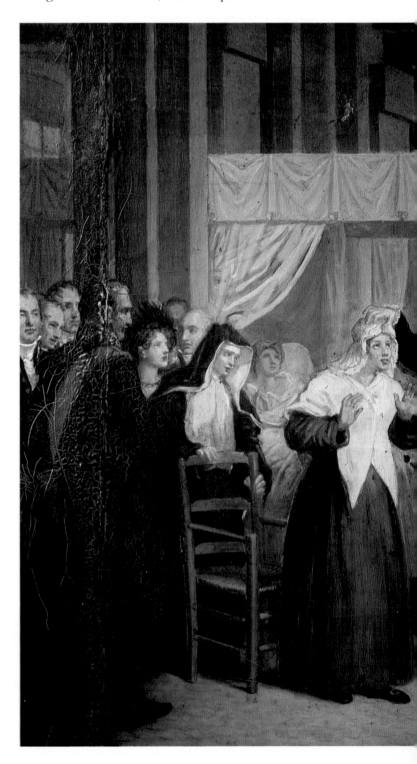

to his knees to wait until called upon to give his symptoms. To the Surgeon-in-Chief of the Hôtel Dieu, the sick poor of Paris were mere material for teaching and study. His colleagues had a phrase to describe the uncaring man they feared so much: "Dupuytren, first of surgeons, but least of men."

This painting, by an unknown artist, depicts a special day at the Hôtel Dieu. Dupuytren, whose usual attire was a grease-stained green coat and filthy boots, is all dandied up for a visit by Charles X, whose brief reign of six years would end in the July Revolution of 1830, the result of his autocratic attempt to restore the old monar-chy. Charles, surrounded by courtiers, appears to be much taken with Dupuytren's demonstra-tion of a patient who has undergone a successful cataract operation. Pressing with his thumb, the uncaring surgeon grips the patient's forehead to make his result more visible, while she ineffec-tually gestures with her outturned palms. In this glittering company, Dupuytren, by then a baron and First Surgeon to the King, cared less about ordinary people than ever before.

Colorplate 33. Musée Carnavalet, Paris.

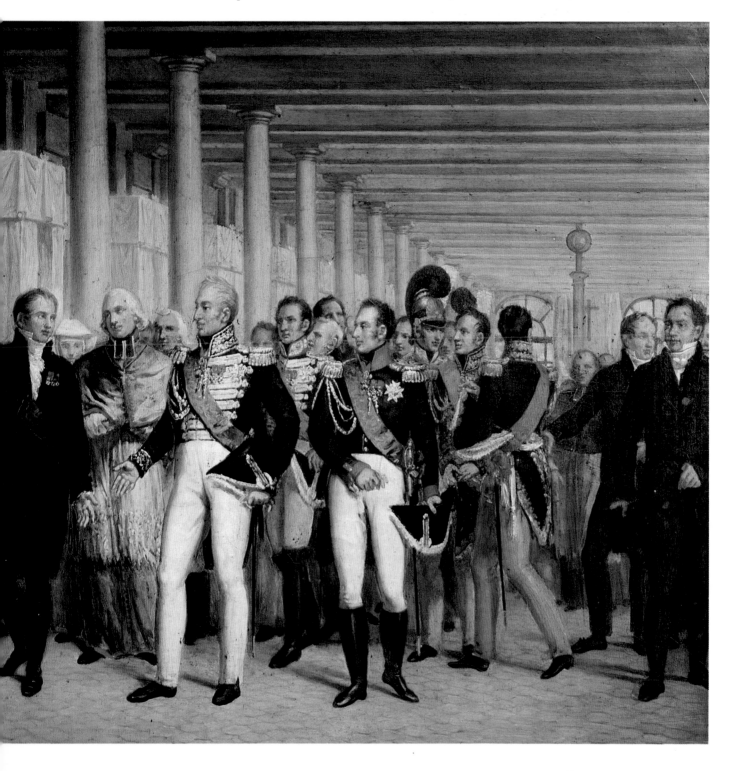

WILLIAM HARVEY PRESENTING A DEER HEART TO HIS KING

1848

Robert Hannah

It has correctly been said that William Harvey's discovery of the circulation of the blood in 1628 was the greatest gift that one man ever made to the ancient art of healing. Not only did his contribution solve a puzzle that had eluded all previous investigators, but it served also as a model of the way in which the experimental method might be employed as the most valuable tool of research into the mysteries of nature.

William Harvey coined an intriguing term for those mysteries. He called them "Nature's closet secrets," and he strove all his life to expose them to the scrutiny of his fellow physicians. The key to his success was the experiments he did on animals. By painstaking observation of the slowly contracting hearts of snakes and other cold-blooded creatures, he was able to make perceptive observations of the various movements of cardiac muscle. He measured the heart's output and noted the way in which the various chambers filled and emptied, and he analyzed the role of the major arteries. He took care to learn the action of the cardiac valves and the contribution of the elastic walls of the arteries as they respond to the heart's expulsion of blood into them. Again and again, he demonstrated how the valves within the veins function to keep blood moving in a central direction back toward the heart.

When Harvey had correlated all the observations and data, he stated his conclusion in the fourteenth chapter of his book, *On the Motion of the Heart and Blood in Animals*, published in 1628. The chapter is only one paragraph in length, but endless in significance. Prior to its writing, the old Galenic theory held sway:

> The blood is constantly being manufactured in the liver, from ingested food. It is then, perhaps by a mechanism of ebb and flow, sent out via the veins to drench the tissues like some ceaseless irrigation system, always being replenished from the liver as it is being soaked up.

To this unsubstantiated dogma, Harvey responded with the thunderous words of the last two sentences of his fourteenth chapter:

> It must therefore be concluded that the blood in the animal body moves around in a circle continuously, and that the action or function of the heart is to accomplish this by pumping. This is the only reason for the motion and beat of the heart.

Harvey was a great favorite of his most eminent patient, King Charles I, who had displayed considerable interest in his research. The king being a frequent hunter, invited Harvey to dissect some of the deer killed in the royal parks. The King was much taken with Harvey's demonstrations. In this painting by Robert Hannah, Harvey shows a dissected deer heart to his sovereign. The boy on the right is destined to be the so-called Merry Monarch, Charles II, who ruled during the Restoration, after the exile necessitated by the Puritan Commonwealth that followed his father's execution in 1649.

Colorplate 34. Oil on canvas. 31¼ × 36" (81 × 91 cm). Reproduced by permission of the Royal College of Physicians of London.

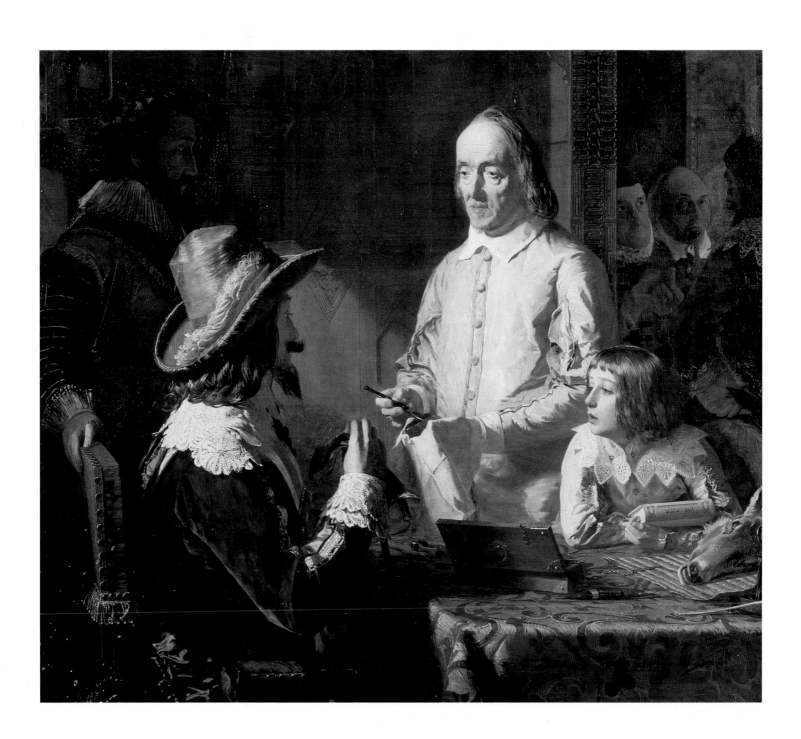

AMPUTATION BY PETER PARKER

Mid–nineteenth century

Lamqua

The art of medical illustration has a long and colorful history. It is probable that the two great anatomists of Hellenic Alexandria, Herophilus and Erasistratus, were using drawings to illustrate their lectures as early as the fourth century B.C. After the Renaissance, when anatomists and artists began to work in close collaboration, the skills of a good illustrator became increasingly essential to the accurate representation of human structure. When the study of disease became scientific and systematized in the nineteenth century, the artist's attention turned more specifically to the depiction of pathological conditions, with the result that some of the drawings done since that time are true works of art despite the sickness they portray.

When the American missionary-physician Peter Parker went to China in 1834, he had the good fortune to be approached by an artist named Lamqua, who offered to paint for him, free of charge, in gratitude for all he was doing for the people of Canton (Guangzhou), where he had organized a small hospital. Lamqua painted in the Western style, having come under the influence of the Irish painter George Chinnery. In fact, there was a distinctly Rembrandtesque quality to his work.

Parker eventually brought back to America one hundred ten oil portraits of his patients. The two presented here are the only examples of the before and after in his collection. Parker's case reports provide the details of the clinical history.

The patient was Po Ashing, a twenty-three-year-old man who, in a fall from a house, had broken his left humerus, the long bone of the upper arm, six years earlier. Although the bone had knit reasonably well, it was broken again six months prior to his visit to Dr. Parker and had gradually become swollen, painful, and awkward: "The weight of it drew him to one side." Amputation was advised and, the next day, carried out in the swift and dexterous manner that characterized such procedures in the days before anesthesia: "The time did not exceed a minute from the application of the scalpel till the arm was laid on the floor." The specimen weighed twenty-one pounds. The stump healed uneventfully and Lamqua painted a follow-up portrait of Po Ashing to complete the record.

Parker entered into his notes the following comment: "All who were present pronounced the case the most remarkable they had ever seen. The patient is the first Chinese, so far as I know, who has ever voluntarily submitted to the amputation of a limb." That statement has been carefully evaluated by Dr. Joseph Needham of Cambridge University, author of a fifteen-volume work on Chinese science, and he finds no evidence to contradict it. Amputation as punishment had been well known in China, and it had also been employed by military surgeons to complete the removal of already destroyed extremities. But Parker's operation on Po Ashing was almost certainly the first time an arm had been electively removed with the consent of the patient.

Colorplate 35. Oil on canvas. 23¼ × 18⅛" (59 × 46 cm). Photo courtesy of the Harvey Cushing/John Hay Whitney Medical Library at Yale, New Haven.

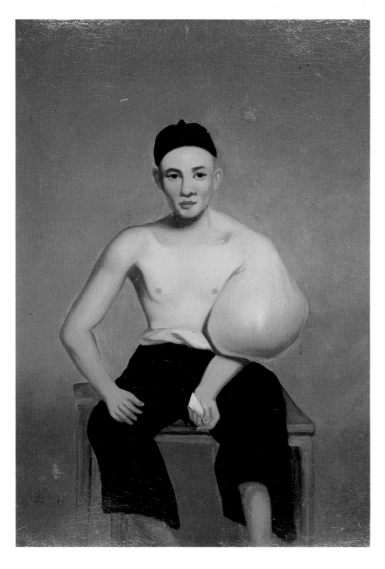 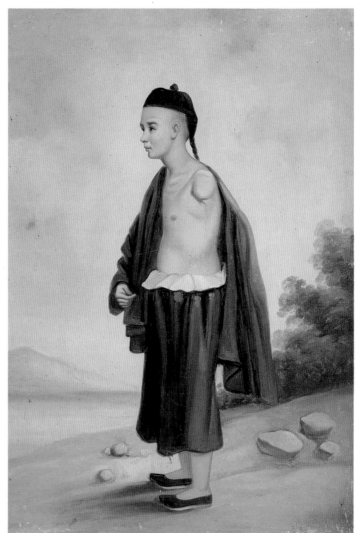

ca. 1837

Honoré Daumier

On July 2, 1823 a tedious five-act melodrama opened at a Paris theater called the Ambigu-Comique, and it was greeted with the deserved opprobrium of its audience, which became raucous in its displeasure. The young actor who played the leading role, that of a serious bandit named Robert-Macaire, decided to attempt a rescue of the obviously doomed play, and he transformed his character into a hapless object of ridicule. The result was so successful that the actor resuscitated Macaire eleven years later, when he wrote a new comedy; the plot involved an attempt by Macaire and another buffoon to outdo each other in acts of knavery and deceit.

Playing the parodic figure Macaire, the young actor Fréderic Lemaitre created not only a popular stage figure but also the inspiration for much of the barbed wit of Honoré Daumier, the great satirist not only of the French establishment but of every aspect of the nation's society. Daumier used Macaire as a symbol in his clever bites at every variety of social target, so that on any one day he might appear as a doctor or a lawyer and on the next as a gigolo or a matchmaker.

Macaire's venue in print was the anti-establishment gadfly newspaper *Charivari*, which each day printed a lithograph and three pages of satiric editorializing. The paper's publisher, Charles Philipon, wrote in the issue of August 20, 1836: "This character remains as the most reliable personification of the period. On the Exchange, in politics, in industry, in literature, and even in philosophy, one discovers everywhere Robert-Macaire and Bertrand, meaning the swindler and his confederate . . . and above all, the excellent collection of sheep ready to offer their backs to the shears of the shearers."

Daumier has as much contempt for the sheep as he did for those who would make off with their wool. In his lampooning of the medical profession, for example, he was almost as hard on the patients as he was on their doctors—and nurses fared no better.

Ironically, he worked at a time when Paris was the center of medical knowledge, attracting doctors from all over the world to learn the methods of the great men associated with the several institutions collectively known as the Paris Hospital. To Daumier, it made no difference: doctors were obvious figures of ridicule in a society whose every aspect was fair game for his sarcasm and vitriolic humor.

In this caricature, the audacious Macaire appears as the big-bellied proprietor of a private medical clinic. Trailed by his retinue of toadies, he grandiloquently asserts: "There you are! Gentlemen, as you have seen, this operation, which everyone said was impossible, has been performed with perfect success." When his followers remonstrate, "But, sir, the patient is dead," Macaire is ready with a typical rejoinder: "It's of no consequence. Without the operation, she would have died anyway."

Colorplate 36. Colored lithograph. 10¾×9" (27.2×23.1 cm). Photo courtesy of the C. C. Fry Collection of Medical Prints, Yale University, New Haven.

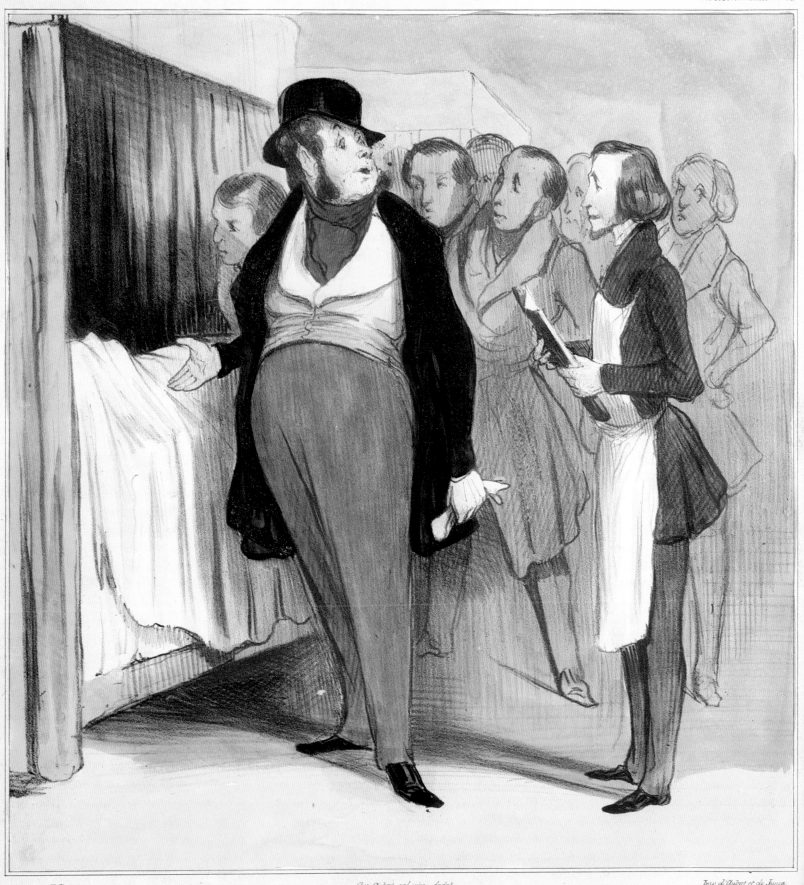

Clinique du Docteur Robert-Macaire.

Hé bien! Messieurs, vous l'avez vu, cette opération qu'on disait impossible a parfaitement réussi... —
Mais, monsieur, la malade est morte..... — Qu'importe! Elle serait bien plus morte sans l'opération.

RUDOLF VIRCHOW

Late nineteenth century
Sir Leslie Ward ("Spy")

Leslie Ward was only twenty-two years old and recently out of art school when he became a regular contributor to *Vanity Fair* in 1873. For more than four decades, he produced a cavalcade of caricatures of British political and social figures that has become famous as an application of the genre in neither a disrespectful nor distorted way. Using the pseudonym Spy, Ward treated his subjects with respect and even a certain amount of dignity.

Perhaps one in ten of Spy's caricatures were neither British nor public figures, at least not in the usual sense. Among those who fell into other categories was Rudolf Virchow the "Pope" of German Medicine. During Virchow's long and productive life of eighty-one years, he transformed physicians' basic conceptions of the nature of disease. His contributions reached their zenith in 1858 when he published his magnum opus *Cellular Pathology*, which enunciated the principles on which medical research would be based for the next century. The first of the principles is the statement that the unit of life is the cell. There is no such thing as spontaneous generation, Virchow emphasized: each cell arises from a previously existing cell. When cells are healthy, the organism is healthy; when they sicken, the organism gets sick. The very title, *Cellular Pathology*, was a statement of the new way of viewing, literally and figuratively, the processes of sickness.

From 1856 until his death in 1902, Virchow lived in Berlin, where he was Professor of Pathology at the University, a leader of the radically liberal German Progressive Party, a member of the Berlin City Council, and, for thirteen years, a delegate to the Reichstag. As a city councillor, he was responsible for vast improvements in the Berlin sewage system, in the organization of hospitals, and in programs of hygiene in the public schools. Every area of Berlin's health benefitted by his activism. At his death in 1902, the *British Medical Journal* stated: "It is not too much to say that modern Berlin is a splendid monument of his zeal in the service of his country."

As if his work as a pathologist, sanitarian, and politician were insufficient to satisfy his intellectual drive, the diminutive bundle of energy that was Rudolf Virchow turned his midlife attention to anthropology, a field in which he produced a total of eleven hundred eighty publications, including several books. When Conrad Roentgen discovered X rays in 1895, the seventy-four-year-old Virchow put them to immediate use in the analysis of specimens that he and his colleagues unearthed.

Virchow's extreme liberalism in public affairs was bound to lead him into conflict with the conservatism and the German supremacist policies of the Iron Chancellor, Otto von Bismarck. The German Progressive Party was a constant thorn in Bismarck's thin skin. Finally, the brawny Junker, skilled in the use of pistols and swords, challenged the bespectacled little professor to a duel. Virchow responded with ridicule, and perhaps with a shy little smile much like the one we see in the caricature. He offered to accept the challenge, but pointed out that it was his prerogative to choose the weapons, and he demanded that the duel be fought with scalpels. In a final derisive thrust, he sent a message to Bismarck that he considered his own life too important to sacrifice on the altar of the Chancellor's honor. The duel did not take place.

Colorplate 37. Photo courtesy of the Harvey Cushing/John Hay Whitney Medical Library at Yale, New Haven.

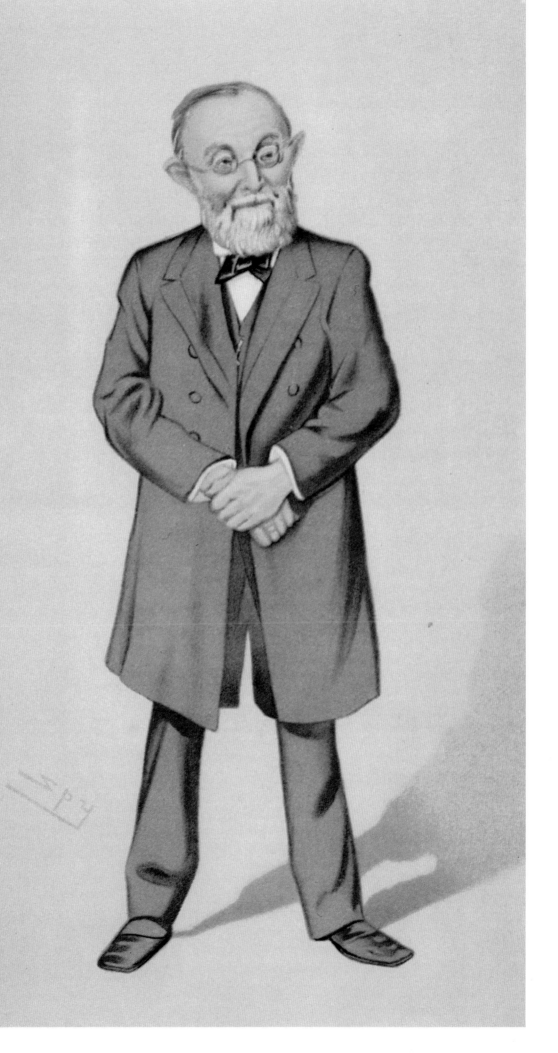

1875

Thomas Eakins

The life's work of Thomas Eakins recalls the illustrious fifteenth and sixteenth centuries, when physicians and artists found benefit in each other's skills. Eakins's keen interest in anatomy is most clearly reflected in his paintings of athletic men in the midst of muscular activity; like his Renaissance forebears, he was fascinated by the human body in motion.

Of his many remarkable paintings, it is generally agreed that *The Gross Clinic* is Eakins's masterpiece. It depicts Professor Samuel Gross, of Philadelphia's Jefferson Medical College, demonstrating an operation for osteomyelitis, a crippling and often lethal infection of bone. The artist himself appears among the observers in the background, sketching the scene. To the right of the surgeon, a woman is seen, work-worn hands thrown over her eyes, cringing to protect herself from the horrifying scene. In those days, a close relative, in this case probably the patient's mother, was required to be present when charity patients underwent operation—a nineteenth-century variety of informed consent.

Perhaps America's leading surgeon at the time, Professor Gross is wearing an ordinary frock coat, as are his assistants, and as is the anesthesiologist at the head of the table who administers open-drop ether anesthesia. The unsterile surgical equipment lies on an exposed instrument case in the foreground, within easy reach of the unwashed hands that will use it. There is no scrub-nurse to pass the few dissecting tools into the palms of the doctors. That is the way things were done in Philadelphia in 1875.

Eakins was revealing much more history than he realized. Nine years earlier, the British surgeon Joseph Lister had demonstrated that wound infections, which occurred after virtually all operations, were caused by bacteria that entered from the air or were inoculated into the incision by the hands and instruments of the surgical team. To destroy the bacteria, it was necessary to wash or spray the wound with a solution of carbolic acid. Using this method, Lister had brought his postamputation mortality rate of 40 percent down to single digits.

Samuel Gross was one of the vast majority of doctors who refused to accept the evidence of Lister's thesis. The principle of germs was too "scientific" for its time, it had to do with such laboratory-born concepts as microscopy and bacteriology, and it demanded a painstaking and meticulous method of operating that was anathema to most surgeons of the period. *The Gross Clinic* portrays a leader of academic surgery caught in an error. It would be a decade and a half before the germ theory would become an accepted principle of American medicine.

Colorplate 38. Oil on canvas. 96 × 78" (243.8 × 198.1 cm.) Jefferson Medical College of Thomas Jefferson University, Philadelphia.

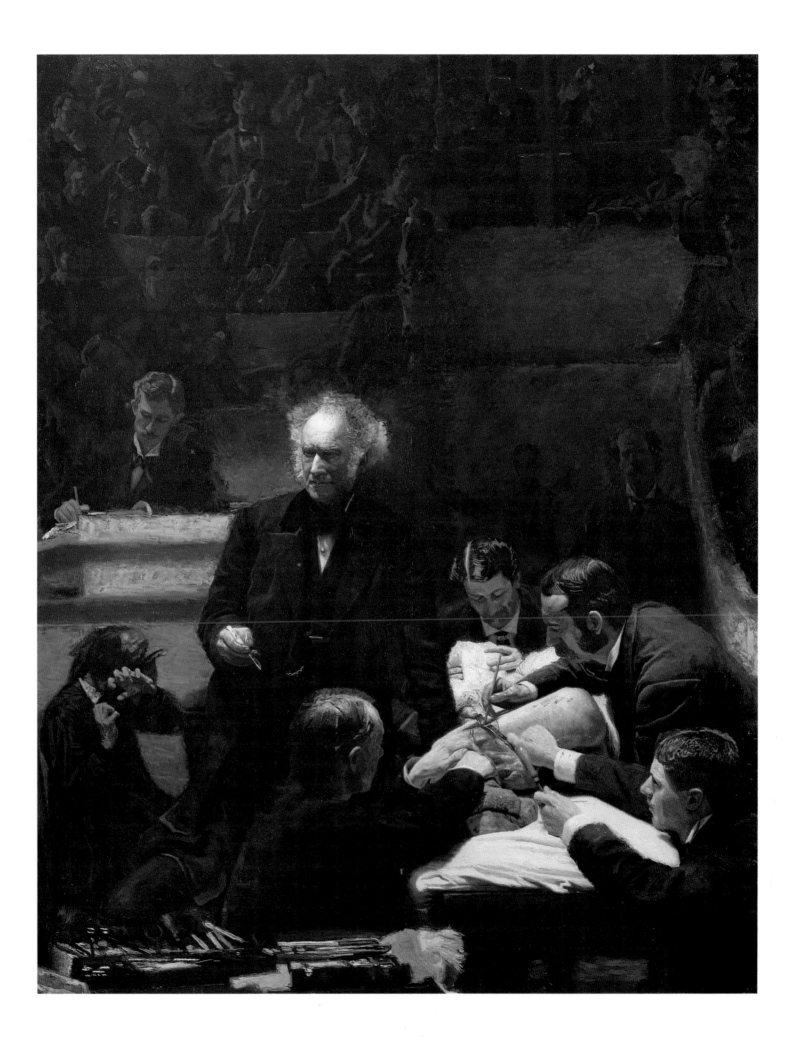

THEODOR BILLROTH OPERATING

1890

Adelbert Seligmann

Just as the hospitals of Paris were the focal point of medical teaching in the early part of the nineteenth century, the German-speaking centers played that role between the 1860s and World War I. Laboratory science took on rapidly increasing importance during this period, and the Germanic universities were the source of the majority of contemporary advances in physiology, biochemistry, pharmacology, and pathology.

Not only in basic sciences did the Germans excel, their clinics and operating rooms were the sites of one major advance after another, as mechanisms of disease and methods of treatment were being elucidated at a rate previously unthinkable. The masters of German medicine were not only grand clinicians, they were also dedicated teachers whose presence attracted vast numbers of young physicians who came from all over the world to work on the wards and in the laboratories. In Paris, the foreign visitors had come as observers; in Berlin, Vienna, Bern, and other great cities they often took part in research and attended formal classes.

No German-speaking hospital was more renowned than the Allgemeines Krankenhaus, the General Hospital of the University of Vienna. It has been estimated that between 1870 and 1914, some ten thousand Americans came to do formal study there. Among the institution's leading attractions was the director of the Second Surgical Clinic, Theodor Billroth. During his twenty-seven years in Vienna, Billroth established the greatest surgical school of his time, and his trainees became the leaders of the field in the next generation. Virtually all the procedures now done in the field of gastrointestinal surgery had their origins with Billroth and his pupils.

Billroth was a remarkable man. In addition to his monumental contributions to medicine and its teaching, he was a skilled writer and a talented musician whose closest friend for many years was Johannes Brahms. Many of Brahms's compositions had their first audience in Billroth's home, and it was not uncommon for the composer to send a score to the surgeon, for approval and suggestions. Two of the Brahms string quartets were dedicated to Billroth. The surgeon's home was a center of music and literary culture in Vienna, in almost the same way that his clinic was a center for surgical progress.

This scene was painted in 1890, four years before Billroth's death, when his health had declined to the point where he was forced to restrict his clinical labors. The artist, Adelbert Seligmann, was the son of a medical historian who was a friend of the Billroth family. The picture's likeness to *The Gross Clinic* is unmistakable; it even includes, similarly, the presence of the artist in the front row.

Billroth came late to the rigid formulas of antisepsis. But as an expert microscopist he well understood the role of bacteria in infection, and he had his own technique for preventing it: his pupils called it "cleanliness to the point of extravagance." The modern aseptic ritual was established years after this picture was painted, but Billroth had already anticipated its major criteria.

Colorplate 39. Österreichische Galerie, Vienna.

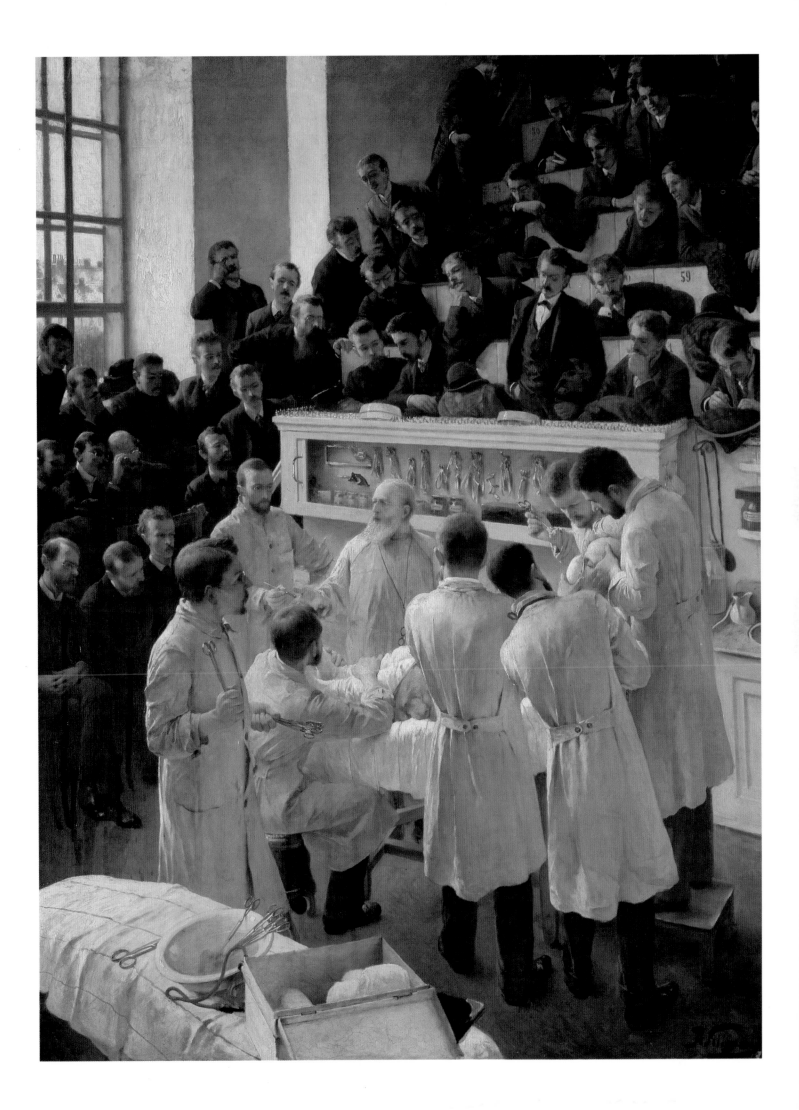

1881–1894

Robert C. Hinckley

The general outlines of the process that led to today's paradigms of medical science and patient care became clearly visible during the second half of the nineteenth century. Four major developments started that process on its eventful way: the invention of surgical anesthesia; the elucidation of the germ theory of disease; the introduction of cellular pathology, by which it was shown that the ultimate unit of healthy and sick tissue is the cell; and the beginnings of modern pharmacology. The first of these developments was a uniquely American phenomenon. As well stated by William Henry Welch, the dean of the medical school of Johns Hopkins University: "The solution of the problem is an exclusive achievement of our countrymen."

The event pictured in Robert C. Hinckley's canvas is one of those thunderclaps of medicine after which nothing is ever quite the same. On the morning of October 16, 1846, John Collins Warren, Professor of Surgery at Harvard Medical School since 1815, was sixty-eight years old and a veteran of almost five decades of the kinds of horror that made torture chambers of every operating theater in the world, not only for patients, but for their surgeons as well. Only a year and a half earlier, a Connecticut dentist named Horace Wells had traveled to Warren's amphitheater at The Massachusetts General Hospital to demonstrate the usefulness of nitrous oxide, or laughing gas, as an agent to produce pain-free surgical sleep. The demonstration failed and Wells was hooted out of the room as a fraud, the perpetrator of what some members of his audience called "a humbug affair."

And now, alongside Warren in the pit of the same auditorium, which from that day forward would be called "the Ether Dome," stood another dentist with another gas. William Thomas Green Morton called his odorous vapor letheon —the term used by Virgil for opium-induced sleep—and by this means he hoped to keep its nature a secret. The patient chosen for the experiment was Gilbert Abbot, a young man with a tumor on the left side of his jaw. Morton, shown here standing behind his patient, administered the ether through a specially designed glass, an inhaling apparatus so new that Morton arrived fifteen minutes late to the amphitheater after a feverish dash from the shop of his instrument maker. In a twenty-five-minute operation, Warren removed the tumor. He would later write that Abbot told him that his only sensation was "that he had felt as if his neck had been scratched." When he completed stitching the incision, Warren looked up at his assembled audience, and in a single short sentence proclaimed the dawn of a new era in surgery: "Gentlemen, this is no humbug."

The new technique needed a name, and it was provided by a man who, although still young, was already being looked upon as a sage of Boston medicine. Oliver Wendell Holmes, thirty-seven years old and soon to be named Professor of Anatomy and Physiology at Harvard Medical School, correctly predicted that whatever name were chosen it would "be repeated by the tongues of every civilized race of mankind." He suggested "anesthesia." In spite of the enormous number of major contributions that have come out of American laboratories and clinics since that time, the invention of anesthesia remains our country's greatest gift to the art and science of medicine.

Colorplate 40. Oil on canvas. 96 × 115" (243.8 × 292.1 cm). Boston Medical Library, Francis A. Countway Library of Medicine, Boston.

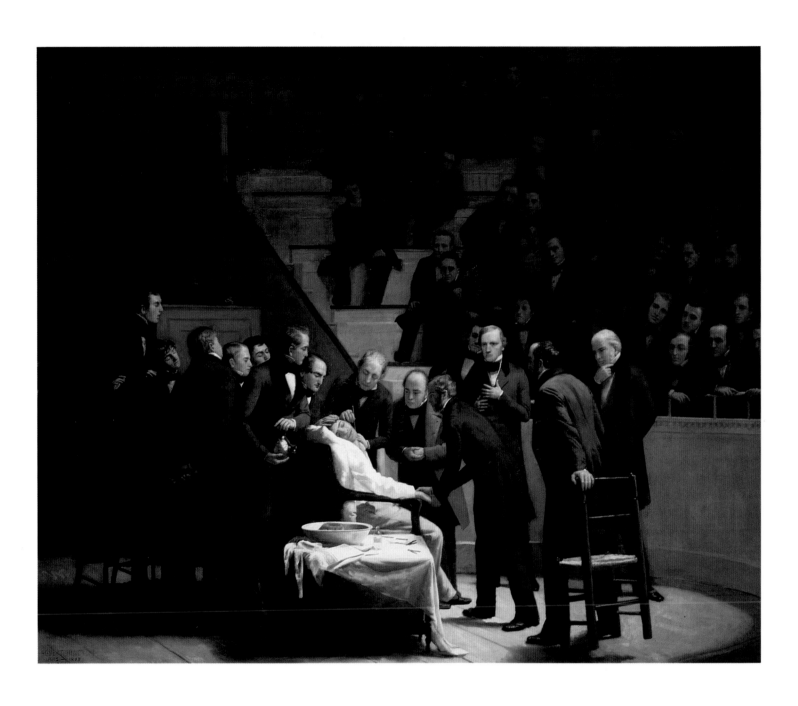

THE DOCTOR

ca. 1891

Sir Luke Fildes

It is ironic that the best known of the many images of healing is the one that shows the medical man at his most powerless. Sir Luke Fildes' *The Doctor* has been seen by virtually everyone, either in physicians' waiting rooms, as part of pharmaceutical advertisements, or in some general portrayal of the solemnity of the profession.

Few would dispute that no one can experience a tragedy greater than the death of one's own child. Fourteen years before Fildes painted his renowned picture of a dying little girl, his son Phillip died in a similar fashion on Christmas morning, 1877. To the painter there could have been no more profound an image of the dedication of the physician to his patient than the one emblazoned on his memory by the diligence and love that the family practitioner, Dr. Murray, gave to Phillip in his last hours. Though he could do nothing to arrest the inexorable advance of death, Murray's comforting presence and his unswerving fidelity to his symbolic role as a healer gave strength to Fildes as his son's life ebbed away.

Sir Luke achieved his stated objective with this great painting: "To put on record the status of the doctor of our time." He somehow managed by his art to convey an aesthetic of life and of death that is perhaps best articulated by yet another revealing comment he made about it: "To me, the subject will be more pathetic than any, more terrible perhaps, but yet more beautiful."

Phillip died at a time when physicians had little to offer their patients, other than themselves, to combat the ravages of diphtheria, scarlet fever, meningitis, or any of the other infectious diseases that carried off so many children. The most they could usually do is what Dr. Murray is shown here doing—keep watch at the bedside and hope that the grim tide would turn, or perhaps that some small crisis might arise that could be survived by a simple measure that only a doctor knew.

The painting was commissioned by the wealthy English sugar merchant, Sir Henry Tate, to be one of the original fifty-seven pictures in the Gallery of British Art whose founding he announced in 1890. A few years earlier, Tate had asked Fildes simply for "an English subject," and the painter immediately decided on *The Doctor*. In an interview which he later gave to a London periodical, the *Strand*, Fildes tells of how he made the sponsor wait four years until he actually carried out his assignment, citing a heavy burden of portrait commissions as the reason for delay. But we may wonder whether the subject, although it immediately sprang ready-made from Fildes' memory (or his subconscious), was not perhaps too painful to start upon until Tate began to press him for the picture. Once he had begun, said Fildes, "It was eventually proved the quickest painted picture I have ever done."

More than a million prints of *The Doctor* were made in the United States alone. The painting was reproduced on a postage stamp in 1947 to commemorate the centennial of the American Medical Association. Things are different now. Though the doctor can do a great deal more, the image has changed. The doctor is increasingly seen as a technologist of space-age biomedical therapy, and many physicians of our time glory in that image. From time to time, it might be well for those of us who are doctors and those of us who are patients, real or potential, to remember the ideal of Luke Fildes: the doctor at his bedside vigil.

Colorplate 41. Oil on canvas. 65½ × 95¼" (166 × 241 cm). Tate Gallery, London. Photo courtesy of Art Resource, New York.

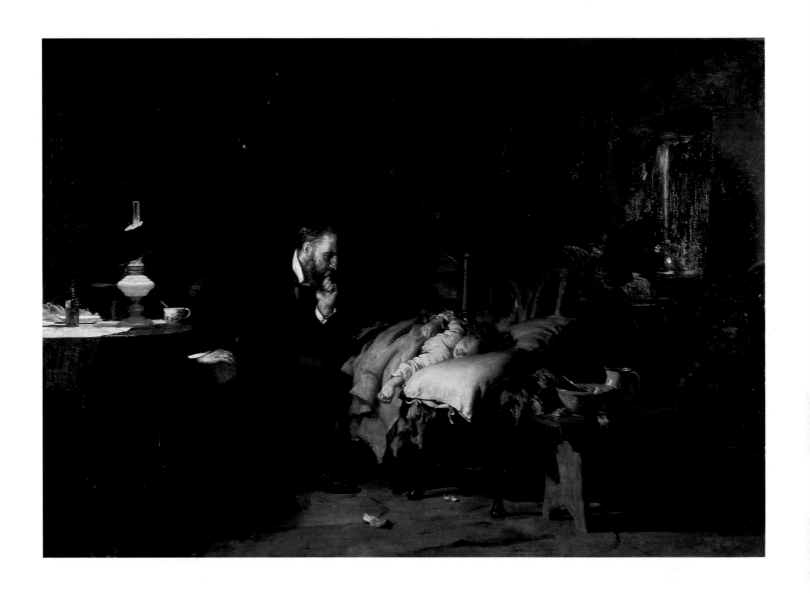

1894

Edvard Munch

In 1803, a twenty-two-year-old French medical student, René Laënnec, described the anatomy of the unique form of inflammation that is the central process in the affliction considered the most devastating contagion of his time, phthisis, or consumption. Using only his powers of observation and a small magnifying lens, he noted the presence in the involved organs of multiple seedlike lumps called tubercles, which grew until they coalesced with each other and destroyed the host tissue.

In 1882, the German bacteriologist Robert Koch, using the most disciplined inductive reasoning and the finest microscopy available, pointed out that the tubercle was the body's reaction to the presence of a microbial invader, *Mycobacterium tuberculosis*. He was awarded a Nobel Prize in 1905.

In 1943, the Ukrainian-born American cell microbiologist Selman Waksman discovered streptomycin, the first effective agent against the ancient scourge. He was awarded a Nobel Prize in 1952.

These discoveries are presented here with a certain symmetry because each of them can be seen as a turning point in medical progress. The identification of streptomycin is part of the establishing of the antibiotic era; the identification of the causative agent of tuberculosis is part of the establishing of the germ theory; the identification of the tubercle as the primary pathology is part of the establishing of the new philosophy of disease.

In replacing the word "phthisis" with "tuberculosis," medical science was expressing its abandonment of the old Hippocratic tradition of naming a sickness for its major symptom because there was no other way. Henceforth, the terminology of disease was increasingly to be based on the nature of the pathological changes it produces in the tissues of the body. *Phthisis*, Greek for 'wasting' or 'decay,' was translated into English as "consumption." There is no better word to describe the destructive effect of tuberculosis during its relentless progression toward an eventual internal decomposing of its victims.

It was Edvard Munch's tragic lot to know about this firsthand. His mother died of consumption when he was five, his eldest sister when he was fifteen. In 1894, when Munch was thirty years old, he began to make prints. Among his earliest is this portrait of lost hope entitled *The Sick Child*. The artist has captured the pallor and exhaustion of the dying girl and the hopelessness of the bowed, grieving mother, already mourning the imminent loss of her daughter. The woman's hat tells us that in a sense her child has already been taken from her, because this is certainly a hospital room. The shadow of the "White Death" of tuberculosis looms over this picture as though to magnify the anguish not only of the mother but of the viewer as well. There is no relief from the inevitability of this child's fate or her mother's despair.

Plate 42. Dry point engraving. 15³/₁₆ × 11⁷/₁₆" (38.6 × 29 cm.) Philadelphia Museum of Art, Philadelphia. Purchased: Smithkline Beckman Corporation Fund.

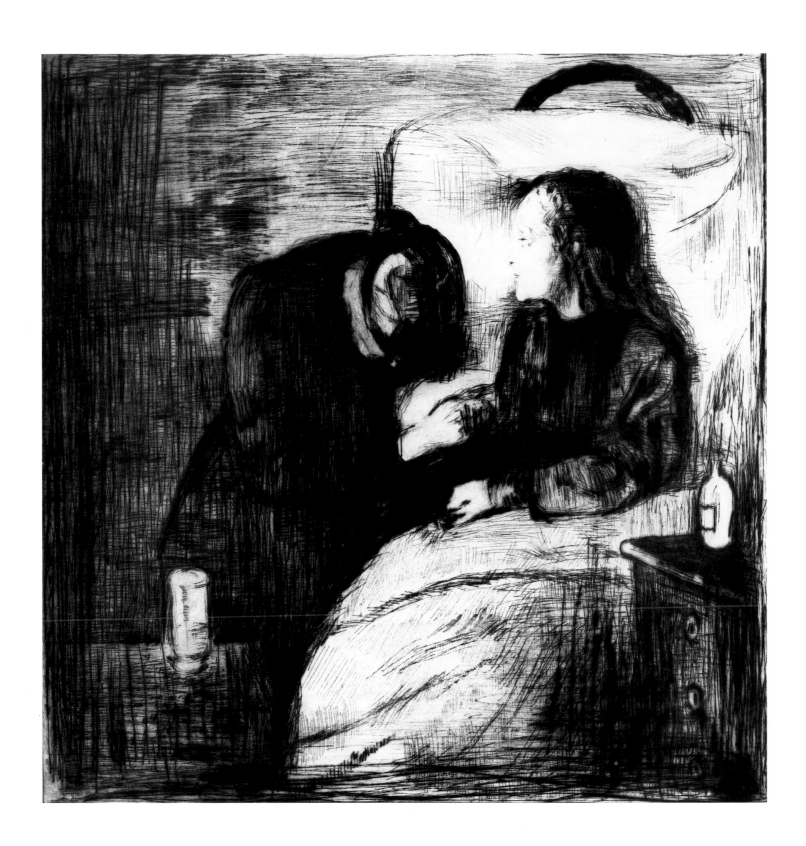

THE FOUR DOCTORS, MEMBERS OF THE FIRST CLINICAL FACULTY OF JOHNS HOPKINS, BALTIMORE, MARYLAND

1905

John Singer Sargent

John Singer Sargent's *The Four Doctors* is yet another of those works of art that are emblematic of a turning point in the history of medicine. This most famous of American medical portraits signifies a series of events that has come to be recognized as a transfer of leadership from the Old World to the New. Even before the medical school of Johns Hopkins University held its first classes in 1893, it was obvious that the bold new experiment in education and clinical care would become the model that all other medical institutions would have to follow if they were to transform themselves into centers of modern research and scientific teaching.

The philosophy of the founders of the school and its hospital incorporated several innovations that were unique in American medical education. For the first time, it was required that all entering students be college graduates. Admission requirements included not only high academic attainment but also satisfactory completion of courses in biology, chemistry, and physics, as well as a reading knowledge of French and German, the two languages in which most of the important contemporary medical literature was written. The new school provided America's first laboratories for students. The medical staff of Johns Hopkins Hospital consisted of faculty members of the school, who were expected to excel not only in teaching and clinical work, but in research as well.

Clearly, the success or failure of the Hopkins undertaking would depend entirely on the quality of the faculty. By a combination of wisdom, luck, philanthropic support, and the magnetic force of an exciting new environment, Hopkins attracted an assortment of laboratory and clinical innovators whom many historians regard as the most talented young biomedical scholars ever assembled in one place. Sargent's magnificent canvas, which can be seen in the Welch Medical Library of the school, pictures the four most renowned of the group as they appeared in 1905: the Professor of Pathology, William Henry Welch, who was also the dean; William Stewart Halstead, the Professor of Surgery; William Osler, the Professor of Medicine; and Howard Kelly, the Professor of Gynecology.

It would have been impossible to overestimate the influence that these four men would have on medical education and patient care, not only in the United States, but throughout the world. Their work and the work of their students, as well as the brilliant contributions made by Hopkins people in anatomy, physiology, biochemistry, and embryology, soon began to eclipse that of the German-speaking schools that had preceded them. By the beginning of World War I, it was generally recognized that American medical science, based on the example of Johns Hopkins, had taken on the position of world leadership.

Colorplate 43. Oil on canvas. 120¾ × 108" (328 × 277 cm). Johns Hopkins Medical Institutions, Office of Public Affairs, Baltimore.

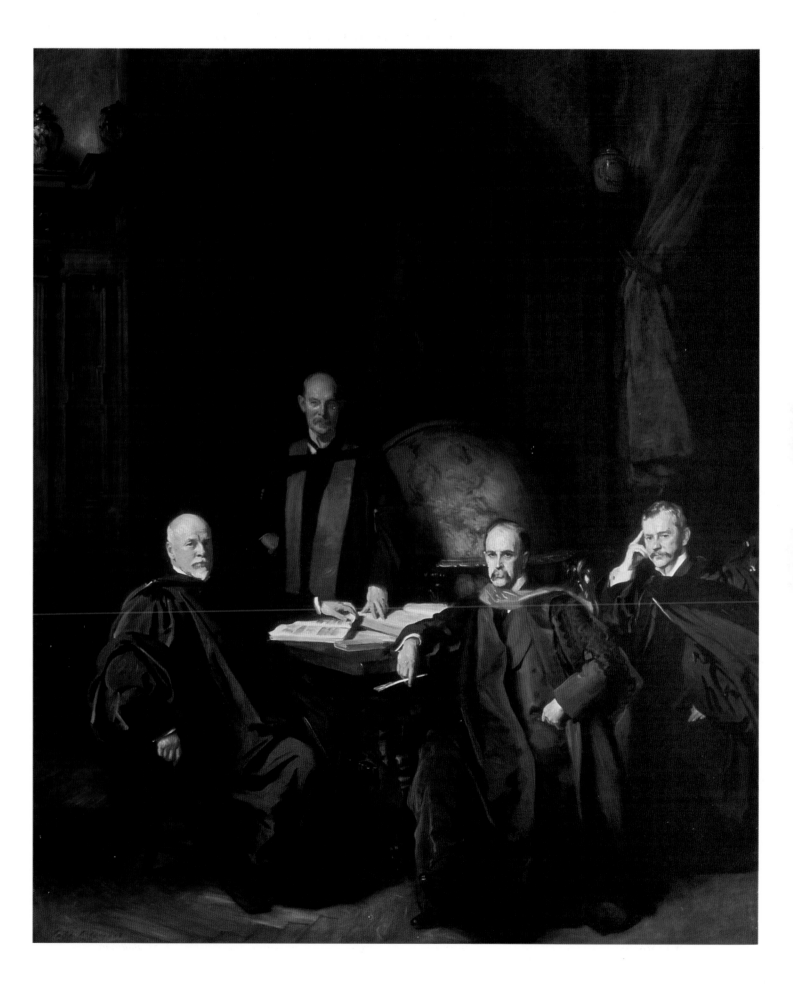

Mid–twentieth century

Ivo Saliger

The German physicist Konrad Roentgen was puzzled by the new form of invisible radiation he had accidentally discovered while experimenting with a cathode ray tube in his laboratory at the University of Würzburg. Because it was invisible and did not reflect or refract, it seemed to him unrelated to light, but he was unable to comprehend its real nature. Stymied, he called his mysterious new discovery *x-radiation*, or *X ray*. In February of the following year, 1896, Henri Becquerel reported to a meeting of the French Académie des Sciences that certain phosphorescent crystals, when stimulated by sunlight, produced rays similar to those found by Roentgen, a phenomenon that was later called *radioactivity* by Marie Curie.

Soon afterward, it began to be noted by researchers working with the new form of radiation that it produced hair loss and redness of the skin on exposed areas of their bodies. There was some destructive effect on biological tissues. As early as November 1896, Leopold Freund of Vienna used the rays to treat a large hairy mole, causing the hairs to fall out. From that point on, progress was rapid in the use of X rays for therapeutic purposes. The first actual cure, of a skin cancer on the nose, was reported in 1899 by Thor Stenbeck of Sweden.

The concept of deep X-ray therapy was introduced in the 1920s. It was during this period that it became firmly established that most breast cancers are highly responsive to X-ray therapy. In this lithograph by Ivo Saliger we see a young woman being treated by this method.

Not much is known about Saliger except that he was born in 1894 and was a painter and etcher of the so-called Austrian School during the Nazi period. At a time when so many gifted artists endured censure and ridicule as producers of decadent and perverted work, Saliger apparently was immune to such charges.

The picture shows the X-ray tube placed, in the manner of the time, close to the breast, a practice that often resulted in serious burns and damage to surrounding tissues, especially in patients unshielded over the parts of the body not being treated. In fact, in this picture there is not even any concession to the patient's modesty, and her entire torso lies naked before the viewer's and the radiotherapist's eyes. The therapist himself is protected by a lead plate, and his radiation-proof goggles prevent us from knowing the exact focus of his gaze.

There is something disturbingly wrong with this picture. The very mystery of radioactivity and its insidious effects on the unwary have often been fuel for the active imagination, and Saliger's lithograph begs for interpretation. Although his overt purpose seems to be a symbolic depiction of the way in which death is thwarted by the X-ray beam, there are glaring (and the word is chosen advisedly) inconsistencies. The chiaroscuro style lights up the therapist and the torso of the perfectly formed young woman, who is hardly the sort of patient who would have been receiving X-ray therapy during that era, when its use in breast cancer was usually restricted to advanced cases. His goggles give the radiologist a distinctly diabolical appearance, and his resemblance, no doubt unintentional, to a pudgy Heinrich Himmler is unmistakable.

Perhaps the symbolism is less overt than it would seem. Put into the context of its time and place, and perhaps its artist, we may be looking at a representation of the Third Reich rescuing virtuous and beautiful Aryan womanhood from the depraved Ausländer—the malignant outsider so despised in Hitlerian theology, who would, like a cancer, enter her body to violate its racial purity.

Colorplate 44. Lithograph. 28⅛ × 40⅛" (72 × 102 cm). Photo courtesy of the C. C. Fry Collection of Medical Prints, Yale University, New Haven.

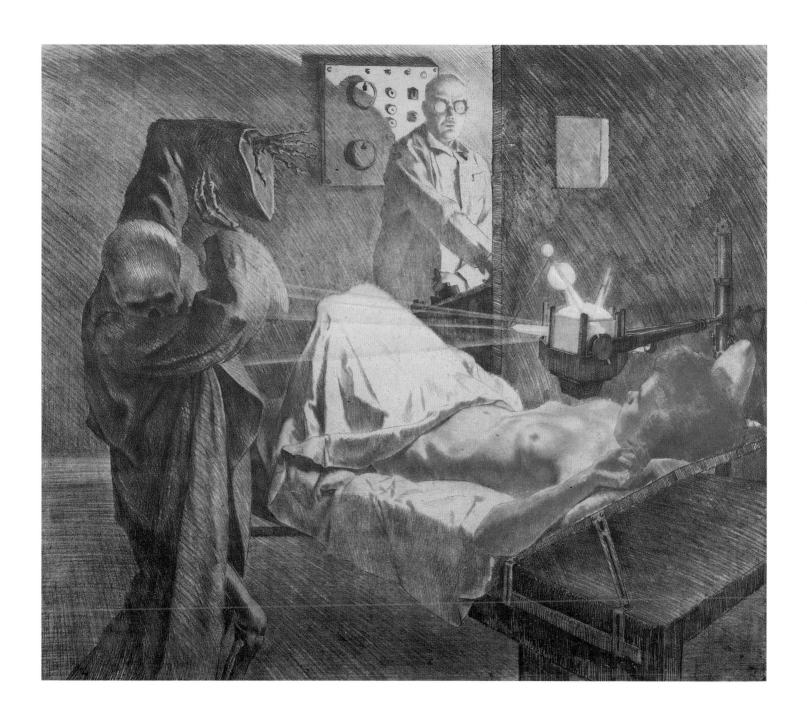

ANATOMISTS,
DETAIL FROM THE HISTORY OF CARDIOLOGY

1943-1944

Diego Rivera

It was the hope of Michael Servetus that the tract he wrote in 1553, *Christianismi restitutio*, would bring about a restoration of principles that he considered to be the essence of true Christianity. Instead, its publication caused the Spanish physician-theologian to be put on trial for heresy in the very epicenter of Calvinism, Geneva; John Calvin himself demanded that Servetus be executed.

Two days after the inevitable verdict, Servetus was burnt at the stake, and every copy of his book that could be found was destroyed; only three single volumes were later found. The unexpected result of his sacrifice was that he became forever enshrined, not so much as a victim of religious intolerance, but as a symbol of the church's relentless war on scientific discovery. Although the heresy of Servetus was theological, the burned book is remembered for the small section in which its author describes his identification of the so-called lesser circulation, the pathway by which the right ventricle of the heart forces blood that has returned to it from the veins around the circuit to the lungs and back again to the left side, so that the bright-red oxygenated fluid can be pumped out to the rest of the body. Long after his theology was a dim memory, the medical discovery of Michael Servetus remained his lasting monument.

Diego Rivera, in this section called *Anatomists* from a fresco on the history of cardiology he completed at Mexico City's Institutio Nacional de Cardiologia Ignacio Chavez in 1944, depicts Servetus at the stake, dominating the figures of medical innovators who made major contributions to the understanding of heart and lung diseases. The unifying image of the dying man aflame in the midst of his burning volumes is made even more horrible by the grotesquery of raging righteousness seen in the figures of the ranting churchmen. The painter is reminding those who think for themselves that danger is never far off.

Seen just to the right of Servetus's inquisitors is the great William Harvey, who in 1628 brought forth his monumental description of the experiments that led him to his discovery of the circulation. The only gap in Harvey's reasoning was his inability to demonstrate the pathway by which blood passes from the tiniest arteries into the tiniest veins. He hypothesized that there must of necessity be what he called "pores," which were shown in 1660 to be, in fact, microscopic passages called capillaries. The man who found the capillaries is Marcello Malpighi, pictured to Harvey's left. Above the head of Malpighi is seen a man lightly knocking on the chest of a young female patient. This is Leopold Auenbrugger, whose childhood experiences as the son of an innkeeper had taught him that thumping on empty or partially filled beer barrels produces quite different sounds than the dull notes emitted by those kegs not yet tapped of any of their contents. He used this knowledge to develop the method of physical examination called percussion, in which the physician raps lightly on the back of one finger of his flattened hand placed on the patient's chest to interpret the characteristic sounds of health and disease in underlying structures.

Above Auenbrugger and appropriately close to the flames is the inventor of the stethoscope, René Laënnec, himself a martyr of sorts, albeit to his own studies of tuberculosis. Not surprisingly, both Auenbrugger and Laënnec, those innovators with sound and pitch, were amateur musicians. The scowling Josef Skoda stands imperiously above them, finger extended heavenward, as if to point out that it was he who codified, categorized, and correlated the physical examination of the chest with the pathological changes that could be identified within.

Every discoverer in Rivera's cavalcade of history stands within reach of the scorching heat of that lethal fire that is the memory of Michael Servetus and his attempt to defy his censors.

Colorplate 45. Fresco (one of two panels). 228¼ × 158⅛" (600 × 405 cm). Instituto Nacional de Cardiologia Ignacio Chavez, Mexico. Photo courtesy of the Detroit Institute of Art, Detroit.

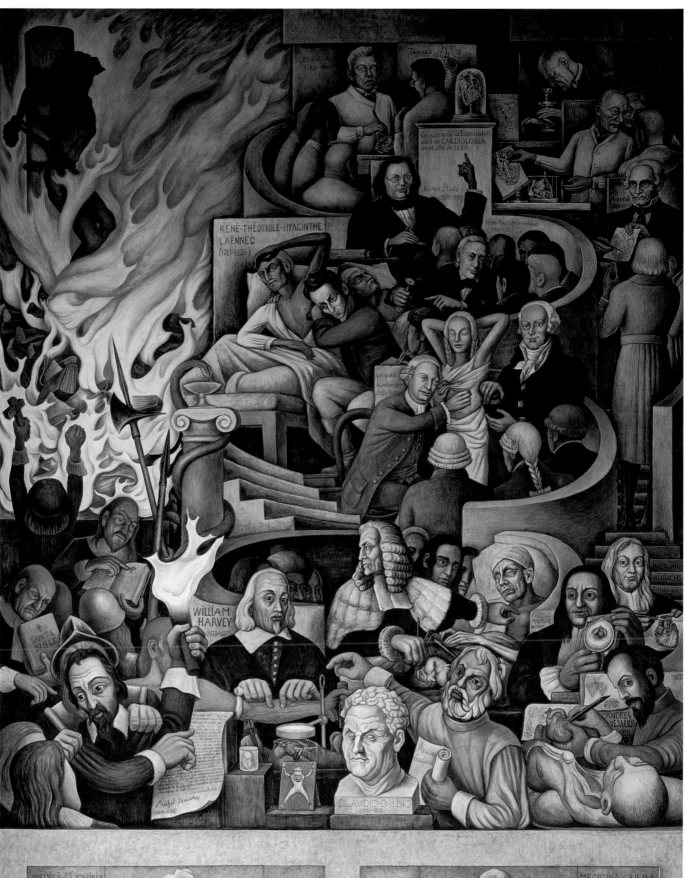

RENÉ-THÉOPHILE-HYACINTHE
LAËNNEC
(1781-1826)

Creación de la Especialidad de CARDIOLOGÍA en el año de 1839

Joseph Škoda (1805-1881)

Jean Baptiste Bouillaud (1796-1881)

Leopold Auenbrugger (1722-1809)

MORGAGNI

RAYMOND VIEUSSENS (1641-1716)

WILLIAM HARVEY (1578-1657)

SAINTE BIBLE

MARCELLO MALPIGHI

Andrea Cesalpino

CLAVDIO GALENO

ANDRES VESALIUS

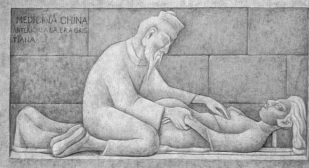

MEDICINA CHINA
ANTERIOR A LA ERA CRISTIANA

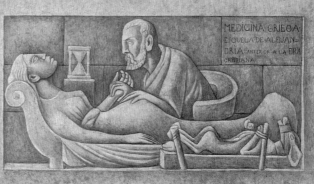

MEDICINA GRIEGA
ESCUELA DE ALEJANDRIA ANTERIOR A LA ERA CRISTIANA

1949

Andrew Wyeth

Of an artist whose creativity had been an inspiring influence on his work since adolescence, Andrew Wyeth once said: "Above all, I admired the graphic work of the northern Renaissance genius Albrecht Dürer. . . . He was discovering the truth, and wanted to put it down just as it was. That's why it has this marvelously *awkward* quality. He was searching." In discussing one of Dürer's watercolors, Wyeth added: "The mundane, observed, became the romantic."

These are observations about another artist, but they seem autobiographical in their perceptive insights into Wyeth's own sources of power. Moreover, in the words of James Duff, director of the Brandywine River Museum (that breathtaking repository of the brilliance of three Wyeth generations): "[Andrew Wyeth] has chosen to paint almost exclusively those who have endured a harsh existence through difficult perseverance. These are strong (Wyeth would say 'tough') people, alone but not obviously lonely, who understand and take pride in their own worth, abilities and limitations."

Margaret Handy was certainly one of those strong people, with pride in the perseverance that had brought her to a rewarding life as a highly respected, dedicated pediatrician. When Dr. Handy graduated from medical school in 1916, she did not have many female colleagues, because the great majority of universities believed that women were not fit to have equal access to a medical career. Yale did not accept its first female medical student until 1916; Harvard would not do so until 1945.

But the medical school at Johns Hopkins University was different. There women were accepted on the same basis as men. The Hopkins leadership, all male, had to be dragged unwilling to this policy, but they had little choice. The embryonic school had almost died aborning, being short of funds by some $500 thousand and unable to complete its preparations to begin classes. A group of four young Baltimore women came to the rescue; among their few conditions was a guarantee that female applicants and students would be on equal terms with men. The university was forced to agree, and the school opened as a coeducational institution in October 1893.

The opportunities at Hopkins were wide open for determined women "who take pride in their own worth, abilities and limitations." It was there that Margaret Handy applied and was accepted. She was twenty-seven years old when she graduated and began her training as a pediatrician. She would settle in Wilmington, Delaware, where, at the time this picture was painted, she was one of only six certified specialists in the diseases of children. All the others were men.

In 1949, Andrew Wyeth's young son Nicholas became extremely ill, and Margaret Handy, through her skill and tireless attention, brought him safely through his sickness, driving out to the family home at Chadds Ford at any hour of the day or night. The boy's admiring father painted two images of Dr. Handy. In one, she is thoughtful, with just a hint of the fatigue and weariness with which she carries her professional burdens. In the other study, we see how in the artist's hands "the mundane, observed, became the romantic": the children's doctor is striding toward her car, on to the next child who needs her. It is night, but the moon is full, in promise of renewal.

Colorplate 46. Tempera on panel. 26 × 25" (66 × 63.5 cm). Brandywine River Museum, Chadds Ford, Pennsylvania. The Betsy James Wyeth Fund.

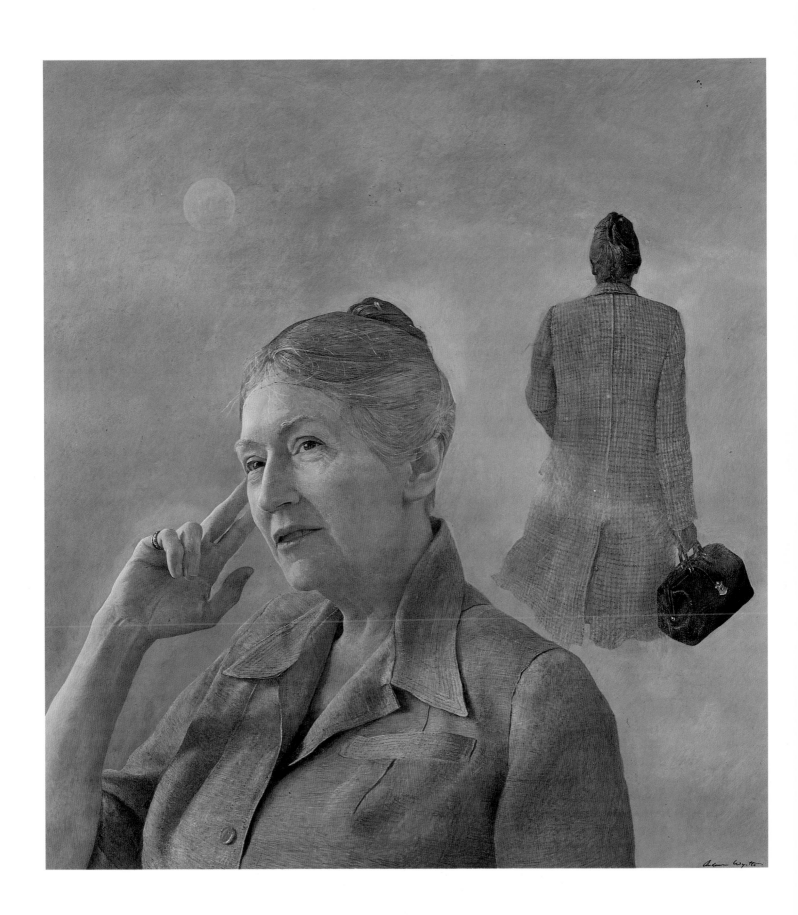

Second Year: Introduction to Clinical Diagnosis, From *The Art of Learning Medicine*

1974

May Lesser

No matter the dazzling accomplishments of today's technological diagnostic methods, the time-honored principles of good history-taking and careful physical examination will always be the basic steps in beginning the evaluation of a patient's symptoms. Neither acronyms like MUGA and CAT, nor corporate-sounding initials like MRI, will ever replace the simple principles of looking, listening, feeling, and tapping—observation, auscultation, palpation, and percussion.

In addition to their value in diagnosis, each of the four techniques has the added advantage of enhancing the physical interaction between the person who is sick and the person who would cure him or her. The laying-on of hands can be a major ingredient of the doctor-patient relationship, a therapeutic encounter that cures far more illness than laboratory scientists have ever been willing to admit. On some level, every patient and every doctor knows about this. Perhaps that shared knowledge explains why it is that medical students still approach their course in clinical diagnosis as though it were a rite of passage, like the first cadaver dissection, the first blood-drawing, and the first night on call. In recognition of its importance, the custom has arisen in many schools that the principles of physical examination are taught by senior members of the faculty and experienced physicians from the surrounding community. Many of the faculty of such courses consider it the highlight of their teaching experience.

To bring life to the freshman year, many medical schools have instituted a program in which students begin to learn about the physical examination shortly after starting their preliminary courses in anatomy, physiology, biochemistry, and the other basic sciences, which take up most of the first two years of the curriculum. May Lesser's painting depicts a freshman class beginning to study in this way.

In the early 1970s, Mrs. Lesser followed a class of students through its entire four-year course, painting and drawing their activities as they progressed. In this picture, she shows a class being taught by the associate dean of the school, who is a specialist in internal medicine. The students have been practicing on each other; one of them has taken off his shirt and is lying down as though he is a patient. The internist is beginning his demonstration of the proper technique to use when examining the liver. In a moment, he will go to the "patient's" right side and gently place his fingers just below the rib margin. On request, the patient will then take a deep breath, to allow his examiner to determine the shape of the lower border of the liver.

Colorplate 47. Color dry-point engraving. 8 × 9" Reproduced by permission of the artist.

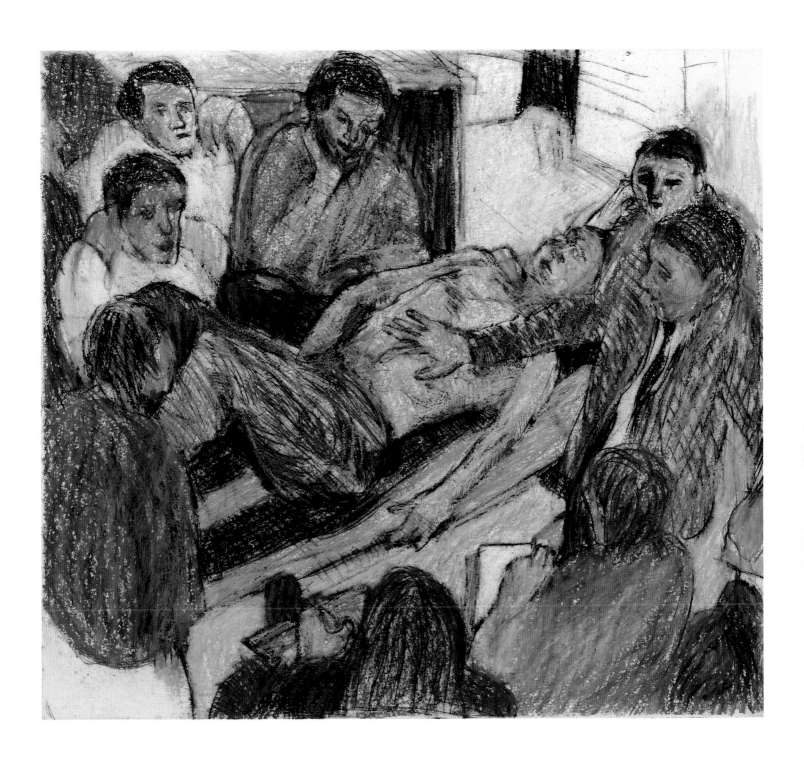

ca. 1975

In a military graveyard of the northeast China city of Shihchia Chuang stands a marble tomb built at the direction of Mao Tse-Tung. In it are buried the remains of a Canadian doctor whose memory is venerated by the people of China, for he was one of the truly legendary heroes in the creation of the People's Republic.

Norman Bethune, a thoracic surgeon on the faculty of McGill University, came from a family in which conscience and obligation were almost genetic. His father and mother were ministers and his grandfather had been a founder of the Trinity College Medical School in Toronto. As a young man, Bethune became increasingly aware of and was outraged by the injustices that the strong have always perpetrated on the weak. Like his parents before him, he recognized that his privilege meant that he owed a debt to those who had less.

Bethune seems to have carried on a lifelong flirtation with his own death. He was severely wounded during service as a stretcher bearer in World War I; a few years later, he developed so desperate a case of tuberculosis that he was not expected to live. It was after his recovery, and perhaps because of that experience, that he decided to become a thoracic surgeon. Bethune never forgot the underprivileged or the downtrodden. During the Great Depression of the early 1930s, he organized a free clinic for unemployed workers, and with some friends he set up painting classes for the children of the poor.

Angered by the Fascist depredations against the Loyalists, Bethune went to Spain in 1936 to join the anti-Franco forces. While there, he organized blood banks and created mobile transfusion units. Within half a year of his return home, he had decided to go to China in order to help in the defense against the Japanese invasion and its attendant horrors. Disappointed by what he saw of Chiang Kai-shek's Nationalists, he met with Mao Tse-Tung and was enthused by the promise that Communism seemed to hold for China. He joined the ragged troops of the Eighth Route Army fighting a guerilla campaign in the mountains between Shansi and Hobei, and there he set up a hospital system and began the training of nurses and orderlies.

Between October 1938 and November 1939, Bethune moved from place to place with the Communist soldiers as they harassed the powerful Japanese army. Driving himself ceaselessly and with very little rest, he accomplished what seemed to his grateful comrades-in-arms to be miracles of healing. His legend among the Chinese grew as his health worsened. His teeth were falling out, he was losing weight, and he developed spells of dizziness, but still he would not, or could not, slow down.

This tapestry was commissioned by the Vancouver timber millionaire, H. R. MacMillan, and made in Shanghai. It hangs in the Sherrington Room at the Woodward Biomedical Library at Vancouver's University of British Columbia. It is a faithful reproduction of a photograph taken while Bethune was operating at a guerilla base in western Hobei. The wraith-like elderly surgeon whom we see is only forty-nine years old.

Not long after this picture was taken, Bethune slashed his finger during a similar operation. He was too rushed and harried to treat it properly, and he developed an infection that he recognized to be lethal. As he lay dying, he wrote in a letter to his commanding general: "The last two years have been the most significant, the most meaningful years of my life. Sometimes it has been lonely, but I have found my highest fulfillment here among my beloved comrades."

Colorplate 48. Tapestry. 78¾ × 63¾" (200 × 162 cm). Woodward Biomedical Library, Vancouver, British Columbia.

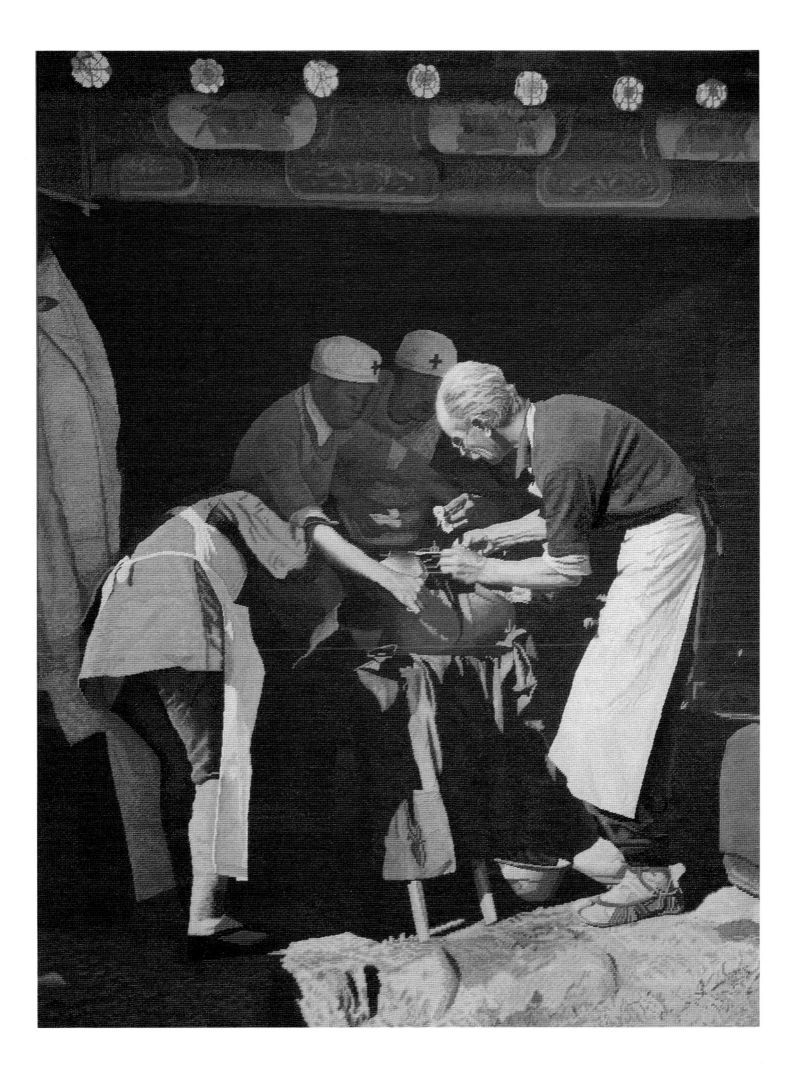